CLIMB WITH CHARLIE

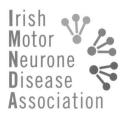 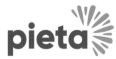

First published in 2022 by
Merrion Press
10 George's Street
Newbridge
Co. Kildare
Ireland

www.merrionpress.ie

9781785373688 (Hardback)

Cover design and book design: edit+ www.stuartcoughlan.com
Typeset in Source Sans Pro

Illustrations of Charlie Bird and Vicky Phelan courtesy of Niall O'Loughlin
Climb With Charlie logo courtesy of Dragon

Front cover image courtesy of Conor McKeown
Back cover image courtesy of Gerry Mooney

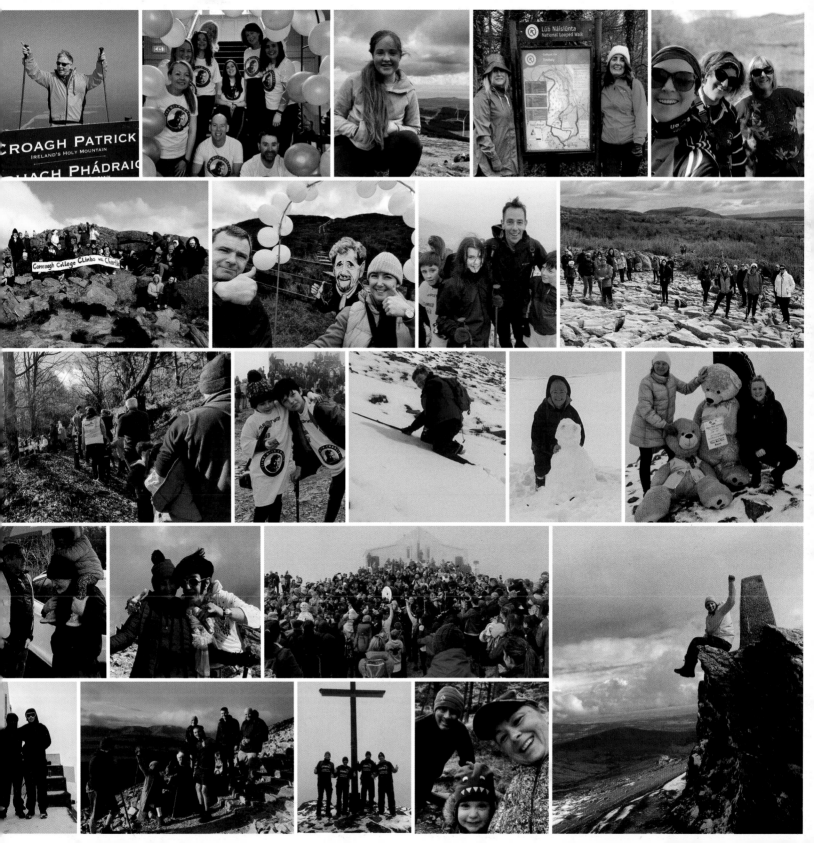

This book is dedicated to those who
have their own mountains to climb every day.
And to everyone who extends the hand
of kindness and friendship.

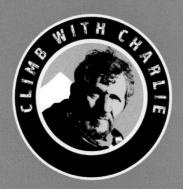

CHARLIE BIRD is one of Ireland's best-known journalists and has had a long and distinguished career in Irish public service broadcasting. He spent four decades working in RTÉ and held various positions including Chief News Reporter, Chief News Correspondent and Washington Correspondent. In November 2004 he was awarded an honorary doctorate of laws by University College Dublin for outstanding services to Irish journalism. In April 2015 he chaired the launch of the Yes Equality marriage referendum campaign. In 2021 he was diagnosed with motor neurone disease and in 2022 he inspired thousands to join his Climb With Charlie campaign.

CLIMB WITH CHARLIE

CHARLIE BIRD

FOREWORDS BY VICKY PHELAN & RYAN TUBRIDY

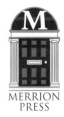

MERRION
PRESS

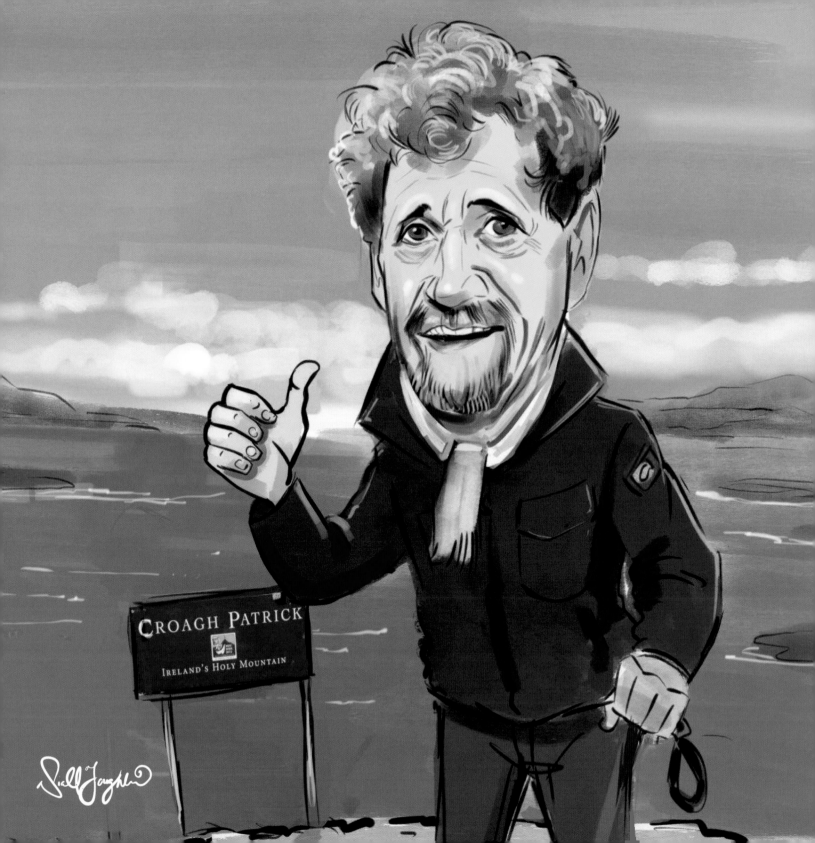

INTRODUCTION

CHARLIE BIRD

IN OVER FORTY YEARS IN JOURNALISM, I have had some amazing experiences and encounters, but in all that time I have never had such a spine-tingling moment as when I reached the top of Croagh Patrick on the Saturday afternoon of Climb With Charlie, 2 April 2022.

As I was struggling towards the summit people were calling out to me: 'Charlie once you hear the music you will know you are near the top.'

I arrived surrounded by my family and friends after almost two hours of stopping and starting – and to be honest, at times finding the going tough as we reached the top of the Reek – and the crowd who had already gathered there to greet me stepped back so I could be welcomed by the forty or so members of the Clew Bay Pipe Band, whose instruments were booming out across the mountain top to the tune of 'Raglan Road'.

The tears welled up in my eyes and I cried uncontrollably, but they were tears of joy. I never imagined in my wildest dreams that I would be climbing Ireland's holy mountain along with thousands of other people and that, in another two hundred and forty locations around Ireland and abroad, tens of thousands of people would be walking and climbing in support of me.

My journey to the top of Croagh Patrick started in late October 2021 when I was diagnosed with the terminal illness motor neurone disease (MND). The same disease that took the life of one of my great friends in RTÉ, Colm Murray, who died in July 2013.

In December I was on *The Late Late Show* with my wife, Claire, and at one point Ryan Tubridy asked me if there was any one thing I wanted to do before my passing. Just off the top of my head I said I would like to climb Croagh Patrick. I had also made the point earlier in the interview that it wasn't all about me, and that many other people were facing difficult times and we needed to help everyone. An idea had just been born. As the show was ending Ryan told me that social media had gone mad and little did I know then that my remarks on the show would lead to amazing support months later for Climb With Charlie.

So here I was now on the top of Ireland's holy mountain with several thousand people coming and going to and from the summit in support of me and, more importantly, the two great charities that I was raising funds for: Pieta, the national organisation which helps people with thoughts of self-harm and suicide; and the Irish Motor Neurone Disease Association, the only organisation of its kind in Ireland which helps people with MND.

One of the issues which had concerned us greatly was what the weather would be like on the day. Initially we had considered two other Saturdays to do the climb and each of those had turned out to be bright, sunny days. On the morning of our climb there was some cloud skirting around the top of the mountain, but eventually it cleared away, giving us a great view of the Reek. Then, when we were halfway up the mountain, the cloud came down again and it began to rain and sleet, so many of us stopped to hurriedly put on our rain gear. But as I reached the top, the gods were smiling down on me, and the cloud parted and the sun reappeared.

There I was, surrounded by my family, many of my friends, and colleagues with whom I used to work in RTÉ. And in a scene that had never been witnessed before, the whole of the Clew Bay Pipe Band, dressed in all their finery, were playing for the first time in their history at the top of Croagh Patrick. As I struggled to regain my composure I was hugged and comforted by Ryan Tubridy and Daniel O'Donnell. Also, by Claire and my five grandchildren: Charlie Jnr, Hugo, Harriet, Abigail and Edward.

Another remarkable moment was when Daniel O'Donnell started to sing at the top of the Reek. After my first appearance on *The Late Late Show*, Daniel, who featured that night as well, stopped me as I was leaving the studio and pressed something into my hands, wishing me well as he did so.

It was a lovely personal gift that he gave me that night. In the days after, we struck up a friendship by texting one another, and when I asked him if he might consider climbing Croagh Patrick with me, he came back instantly and said he would. He was true to his word, and the image of Daniel singing on Croagh Patrick is one that will be remembered for a long time.

Daniel was followed by Matt Molloy from The Chieftains, someone to whom I had grown close since I began visiting Westport. On our first visit, we went into the well-known Matt Molloy's pub and Matt was in there. We started chatting and I asked him if he would climb the Reek with me and he said he would love to. And here was another memorable moment on the day of the climb: Matt playing his flute on the top of Croagh Patrick, a little session starting as the Clew Bay Pipe Band joined in with him.

There I was, surrounded by my family and friends witnessing a little bit of history on the summit of the holy mountain. Among the thousands of other people who climbed with me were former boxer Barry McGuigan and the Chief of Staff of the Defence Forces, Lieutenant General Seán Clancy. All these images were so powerful.

Earlier I had used my voice banking app to deliver my few words to everyone. This was probably a first – someone who had lost their voice using modern technology to address people at the top of the Reek. For weeks I had been thinking of what I would say. I began by saying that the climb was not just about me, but everyone across the country who was extending the hand of friendship by taking part in the hundreds of climbs and walks.

I had promised that I would light five candles at the top of the mountain. Fr Charlie McDonnell, the priest who we had got to know so well, and who, along with Inspector Denis Harrington, had played a key role in helping to organise the climb, arranged for five beautiful candles to be made. Fr Charlie had also made sure that the small church at the top would be opened and that myself and my family could have a private moment there as we lit the candles.

When my immediate family and I entered the tiny church, it was a very emotional moment for all of us. This tiny white church can be seen for miles when the Reek is bathed in bright sunshine. And it looks down on the stunning sight of Clew Bay. It was built in 1905, so as I stepped inside with Claire, my two daughters, Orla and Neasa, and my five grandchildren, I knew in a way I was stepping back in time and history.

A local lady in Westport, Catherine Roddy, had made the lovely candles. The first one I lit was for my friend Vicky Phelan. After her appearance on *The Late*

Late Show in November 2021 I had reached out to her and, a couple of weeks later, Claire and I visited her at her home in Limerick. As a result of that meeting we struck up a friendship. Vicky had hoped to wave me off on the morning of our climb but because of her illness she was unable to travel to Croagh Patrick.

The second candle I lit was for everyone with a terminal illness. The third candle was for everyone who I describe as being in a dark place and people who struggle every day to climb their own personal mountains. The fourth candle I lit was to celebrate everyone who worked so hard to help in the battle against the pandemic. And the last candle was for the people of Ukraine, to shine a light into the genocide which was happening in that country.

I will never forget those few minutes in the church surrounded by my family as long as I live. Even today I find it hard to believe what happened on that Saturday, not just on Croagh Patrick but right across Ireland and in many places abroad. It was a powerful moment, with so many people showing kindness, love and affection and extending the hand of friendship not just to Climb With Charlie, but to all their neighbours and friends. A few people from the Westport area told me afterwards that what happened on that Saturday will go down in the annals of the Reek.

Finally, there was one poignant moment for me on the day. My great pal and colleague Jim Fahy, who had climbed and reported on events on the Reek over many years for RTÉ, had promised to climb with me, but sadly he passed away before he could join me. But his spirit and the spirit of the mountain made the day one to remember not just for me, but for everyone who climbed on that lovely day.

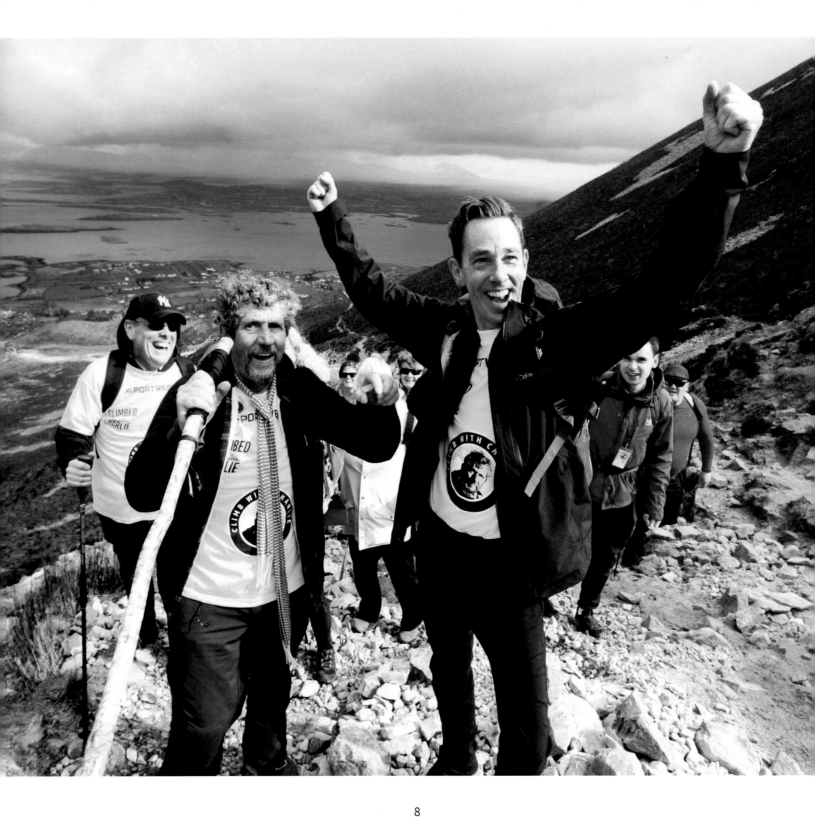

FOREWORD

RYAN TUBRIDY

I'VE BEEN WATCHING CHARLIE BIRD on television for more than thirty years. Even as a young viewer, I understood whatever story he told, as he did so with a clarity and an accessibility that few reporters could hope to achieve. Charlie's boyish enthusiasm and insatiable curiosity earned him the trust, admiration and, ultimately, the love of the nation.

Perhaps it's for these reasons that Charlie's appearance on *The Late Late Show* on 10 December 2021 was so emotional. The Charlie I spoke to that night was a very different man to the one I had come to know down through the years. Here was the iconic reporter with the urgent voice now vulnerable, haunted and in pain.

Like everyone else, I heard and read about Charlie's diagnosis with motor neurone disease with a heavy heart. I have lost some beautiful people to this cruel illness, but it was hard to fathom Charlie Bird being anything other than robust, relentless and resilient, and yet here he was wearing his broken heart on his sleeve on live television.

The first thing that struck me and most viewers was the voice. Charlie's trademark, in many ways, has always been that wonderful voice that spoke in urgent and compelling tones. He might have been in Colombia or South Africa or Stormont telling us all about unfolding events before signing off: 'Charlie Bird, RTÉ News, Belfast!' On that dark December evening, it was hard to contain my shock at how that wonderful instrument had deteriorated as the MND took hold of Charlie's body. We could see the struggle to get the words out, we could sense the frustration at having to make a great effort to do something that was so simple only weeks previously.

The second thing I noticed was Charlie's eyes. He looked shocked and a little horrified by what was happening to him. It was like he was watching 'developments' from within. He was broken-hearted, and it was writ large on his face and in those plaintive eyes. He spoke of how upset he was by the diagnosis and how sad he was at the prospect of a limited life ahead. I watched and listened and tried to process what was happening to this wonderful man. How much should I ask? How much does Charlie want to say? Is it all too much?

Every now and again, I looked to Charlie's left where his wife, Claire, sat stoically. Occasionally, when the moment required it, she would take his hand or touch his arm. Claire was the anchor in this moment and she allowed Charlie to stay strong and press on.

For all the sadness I've described here, I need to mention the other fascinating thing about Charlie. Despite the haunted eyes, despite the weakened voice and despite the pervasive sense of despair, there was the faintest glimmer of the old Charlie, and it was that tiny glimmer of hope that was to change everything.

When I asked a relatively mundane question about what Charlie wanted to do next in his life, he said that he wanted to climb Croagh Patrick. And with that, it all kicked off. We finished our chat, I walked Charlie to the studio door, we hugged, we cried and we both knew that something special could come next.

Within days, the phones started to hop; promises were made and offers were coming in thick and fast.

It was at this moment that the old Charlie I knew was back in the room. The sorrow was replaced by the enthusiasm, passion and energy that have been the Charlie Bird characteristics since he first picked up a microphone. The Climb With Charlie planning had begun and everyone wanted to be part of the story. Daniel O'Donnell was in. Vicky Phelan was in. Baz, Dermot and a host of colleagues were in and, most importantly, the people of Ireland wanted to show their love and appreciation for Charlie Bird.

On 7 January a new, invigorated and excited Charlie joined us on *The Late Late Show* and what a beautiful moment that was. Gone were the haunted eyes and the despondency. Here was a man in love with life, hungry for action and ready to motivate a nation. Charlie and his loyal dog, Tiger, were in flying form that night and it was a joy to watch. In the audience, Charlie's daughters looked on with glassy eyes as they watched their dad address the nation with gusto. Friends and colleagues were there to pledge their support – this was no lonely road.

On a mission to raise funds for the Irish Motor Neurone Disease Association and Pieta, two charities that mean so much to Charlie, the climb was on and the countdown began.

All roads led to Croagh Patrick on 2 April 2022. It was a beautiful spring morning. All over Ireland, and indeed the world, people climbed local hills and mountains in solidarity with what felt like a pilgrimage in Mayo. The ascent was marked by strangers greeting each other and sometimes helping each other when it got troublesome on the steep climb. This was the spirit of the day. Charlie led the march and made it to the top in no time. I will never forget standing with Charlie

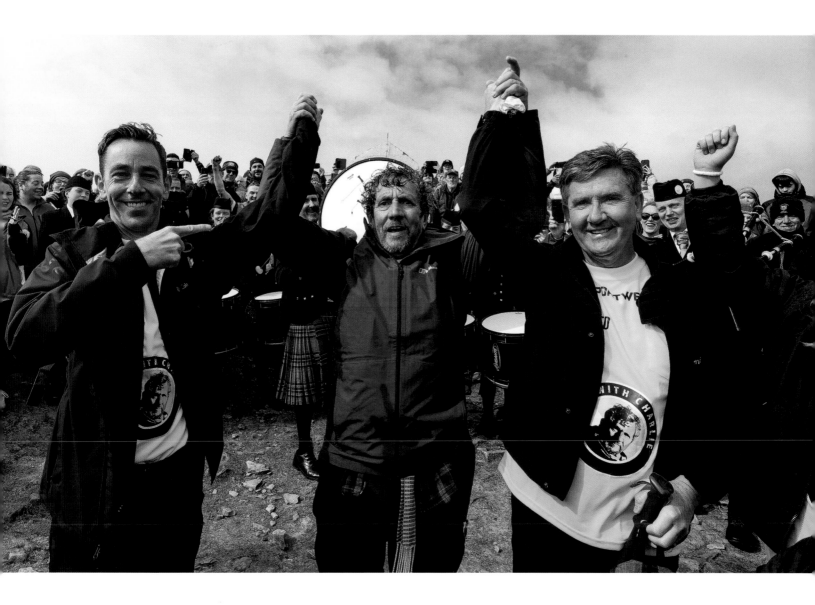

and Claire and all the young Birds gathered around as a massive crowd held their phones aloft to capture the moment. Bagpipes were blown, drums were beaten and the sun came out to complete the picture. Charlie spoke, Daniel sang, everyone cried, and all over Ireland people dug deep to donate over €3 million for much-needed research and resources.

This was a story of two Charlies. It could have gone either way, but the triumph of it all lay and continues to lie within Charlie himself. Something special happened on Croagh Patrick that April morning. The country needed to vent after two dark years. People wanted to participate in and belong to a moment, and in Climb With Charlie we got it.

FOREWORD

VICKY PHELAN

I HAVE NEVER CLIMBED CROAGH PATRICK and, at 47 years of age and terminally ill with cancer, I know that I never will. However, on a beautiful Saturday in April, I came as close as I will ever get to climbing the Reek thanks to Charlie Bird and his Climb With Charlie initiative – one that saw thousands of people all around the country climb, hike or walk a hill or mountain in their locality on 2 April to show their support for Charlie and the many people who climb mountains every day due to their physical and mental-health challenges.

Charlie set himself the target to climb Croagh Patrick and I, along with thousands of others, jumped on the Charlie bandwagon and offered myself up to the Reek. Unfortunately, my body decided not to cooperate and I was unable to make it to Mayo to lend my support. However, my family undertook to make the four-hour trip from County Kilkenny to County Mayo to climb on my behalf. This undertaking was hugely significant, not just for me, but for my whole family.

The weeks spent preparing for the climb distracted my family from the elephant in the room – my deteriorating health – and helped them to have something positive to focus on during a very difficult period with my illness, in which I spent over two weeks in hospice care. Talk of which sticks to bring and what clothes to wear distracted us all from the fact that I was now shuffling around from A to B on a Zimmer frame and in no shape whatsoever to make the trip out West.

My situation galvanised my family further, because they knew just how much it would have meant to me to make it to the top of Croagh Patrick. And so, on the day of the climb, when my family made it to the top and called me from the summit, it was a beautiful moment. We were all so very emotional. There were tears, but they were tears of joy. There was no sadness. I was improving physically day by day and that's all that really mattered. Yes, I would have given anything to be there with my family, with Charlie, with all my supporters at the top of the Reek, but watching my family scale Croagh Patrick and reach the summit on my phone was a very proud moment for me and one I will always cherish.

Throughout that morning and afternoon, I followed friends and followers on Instagram and Facebook and congratulated them on their achievement of reaching the top of Croagh Patrick. As the crowd swelled and Daniel O'Donnell took to the stage to announce Charlie's arrival, the whole summit exploded with emotion like I have never seen before. My friend John Wall had me on speakerphone and handed the phone over to Daniel, who introduced me to the crowd gathered there. A huge cheer erupted. Charlie was standing behind Daniel. Seeing him standing there made me very emotional and I said a few words to thank this wonderful man for making this unique event possible.

It was all very emotional, but the most emotional moment was yet to come for me when Charlie lit his five candles in the chapel. One of Charlie's team recorded the moment Charlie sombrely took out his five candles and lit them for each of his intentions, the first of which was for me. Knowing how much it now took out of Charlie to talk, to see him light my candle and to dedicate it to me using his own voice just made the gesture so very special and meaningful for me. I will never forget that moment.

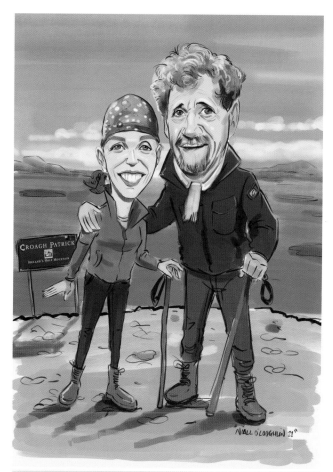

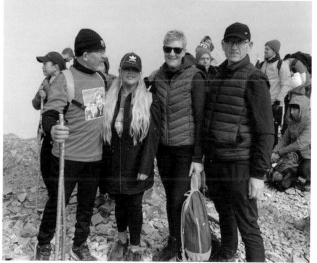

A WORD ON CROAGH PATRICK

HARRY HUGHES

Croagh Patrick, Ireland's Holy Mountain, has been a place of ritual for thousands of years and a site of Christian pilgrimage for the past 1,500 years. It is a stunning sacred landscape that still inspires pilgrims to climb to its summit on the last Sunday of July each year, to participate in the mountain's annual pilgrimage. It is a place of wonderment and myth, history and archaeology.

An archaeological excavation on the summit in 1995 revealed pre-Christian activity. An enclosing rampart was discovered with many hut sites and a sizable building, which was radiocarbon dated to the fifth to eighth centuries AD. The present oratory was built in 1905 and extended in 1961.

It is recorded in the *Book of Armagh* that St Patrick visited the mountain in AD 441. It states in the book, 'And Patrick proceeded to Mons Aigli intending to fast there for forty days and forty nights, following the example of Moses, Elias and Christ.' Croagh Patrick, colloquially called 'The Reek', was previously known as *Cruachán Aigli* or *Mons Aigli*, believed to mean Eagle Mountain. It was renamed in the fourteenth century in honour of our national saint. A corrie on the north side of the mountain is where St Patrick banished the snakes from Ireland.

Pilgrims traditionally performed and revered the Stations, which includes *Leacht Benáin* on the ascent, *Teampall Phádraig, Leaba Phádraig*

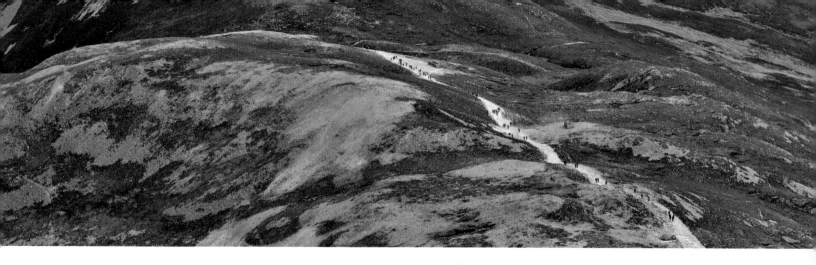

on the summit and *Reilig Mhuire* on the descent. It is Ireland's oldest pilgrimage, and when you set foot on the mountain you are walking in St Patrick's footsteps. Another ancient pilgrim path is the *Tóchar Phádraig*, a 35km walk from Ballintubber Abbey to Croagh Patrick.

In addition to the pilgrimage, for centuries Croagh Patrick functioned as a beacon in the Irish landscape. It is the site of three cosmological alignments. The most famous alignment is the Rock of Boheh, where the sun rolls down the slope of the mountain twice a year, on 18 April and 24 August. The purpose of these alignments is lost in the mists of time.

In 1989, environmentalist David Bellamy joined thousands of locals in protesting against the proposed mining of gold from the mountain. A year later, Minister Robert Molloy decided not to renew the exploration licence as the mountain is part of our national and religious heritage.

Some interesting tales include weddings taking place on the summit, the first being recorded in the 1906; a local hermit, 'Bob of the Reek', being buried on the summit in the 1830s; the poet Patrick Kavanagh calling the pilgrimage 'A Glorious, Singing, Laughing Climb'; and a transatlantic cruise liner bringing pilgrims from the US to Clew Bay in 1928.

Croagh Patrick is Ireland's most climbed mountain, with consequential issues with erosion. In recent years, a team of specialist builders have been reconstructing the path. Local landowners and the parish fully support this initiative. The Reek has attracted many illustrious people, such as President Éamon de Valera, Princess Grace Kelly of Monaco and now the legendary Charlie Bird.

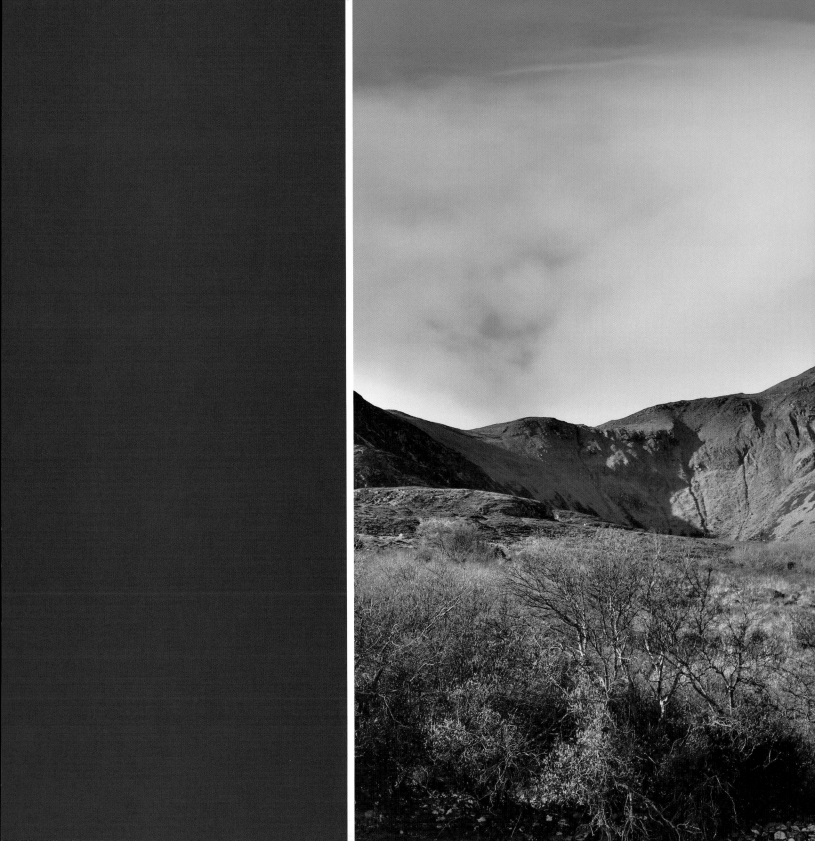

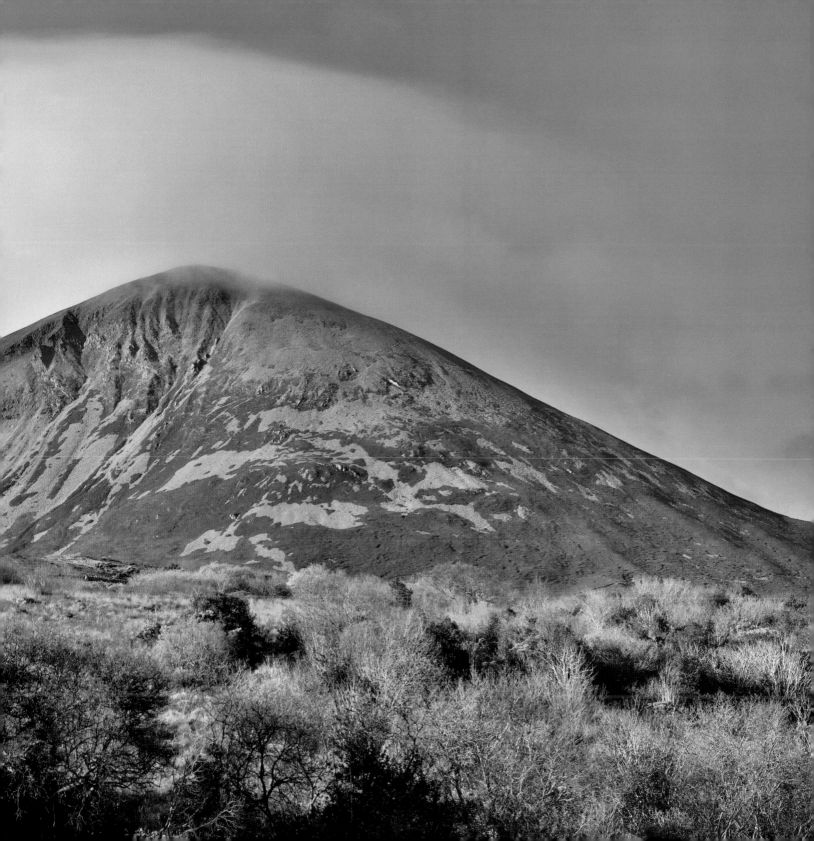

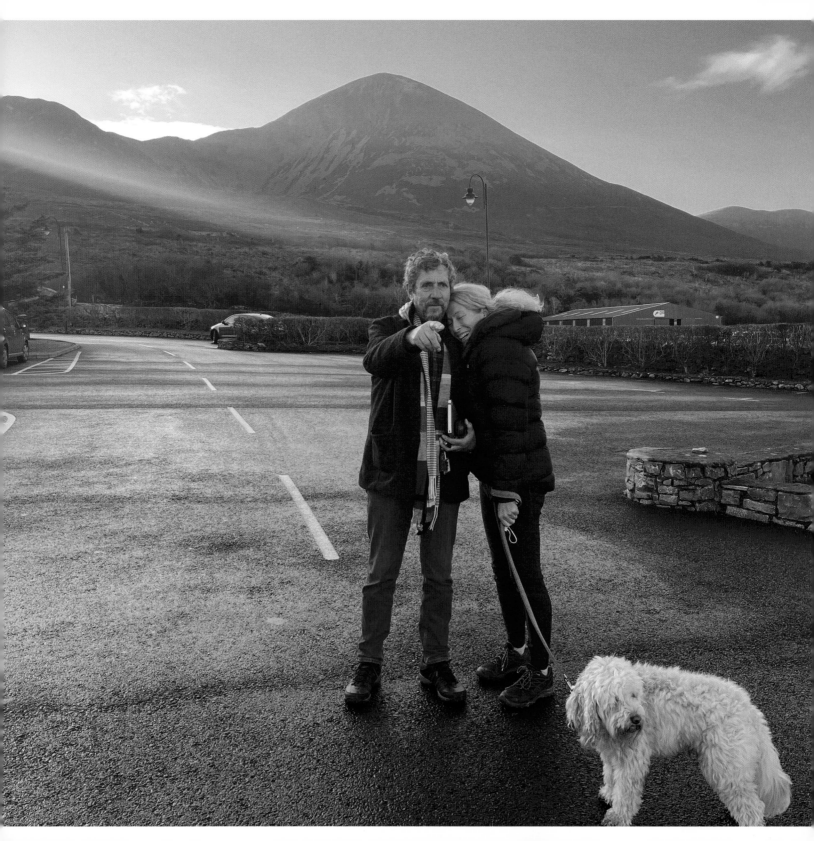

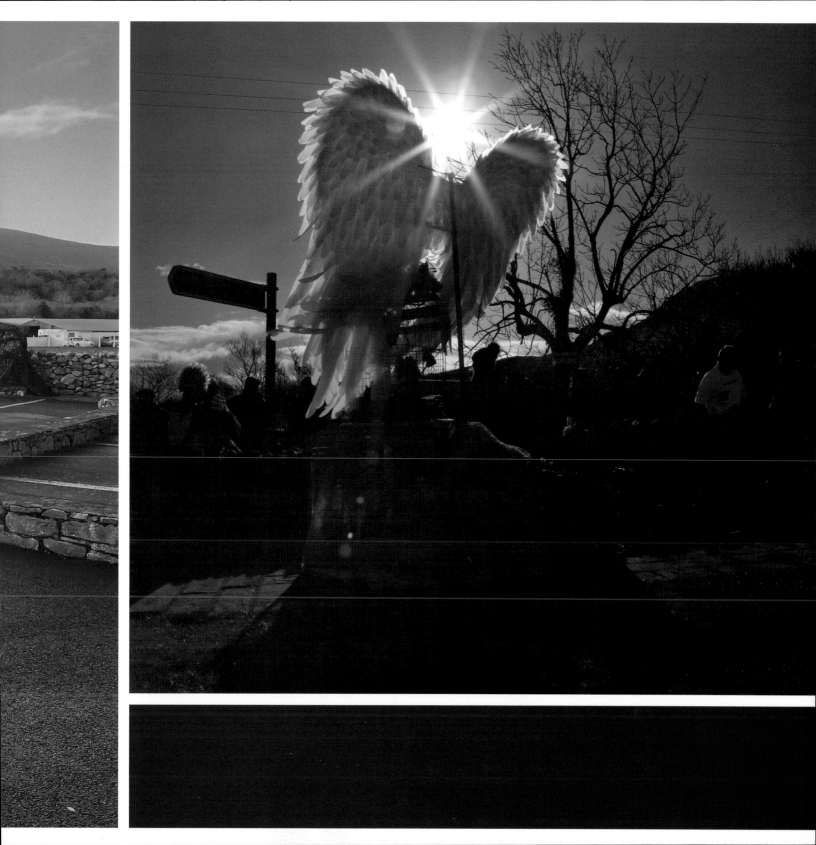

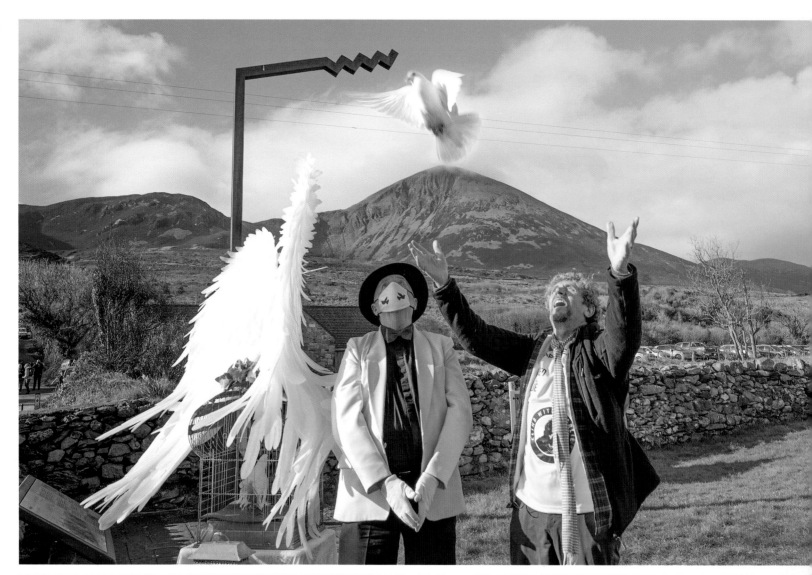

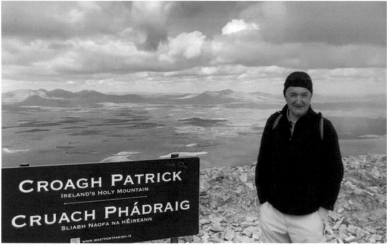

CROAGH PATRICK
IRELAND'S HOLY MOUNTAIN
CRUACH PHÁDRAIG
SLIABH NAOFA NA hÉIREANN
WWW.WESTPORTPARISH.IE

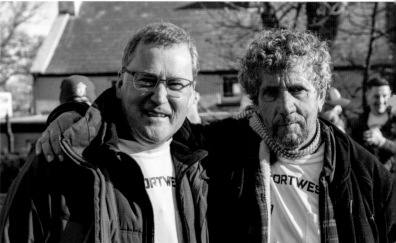

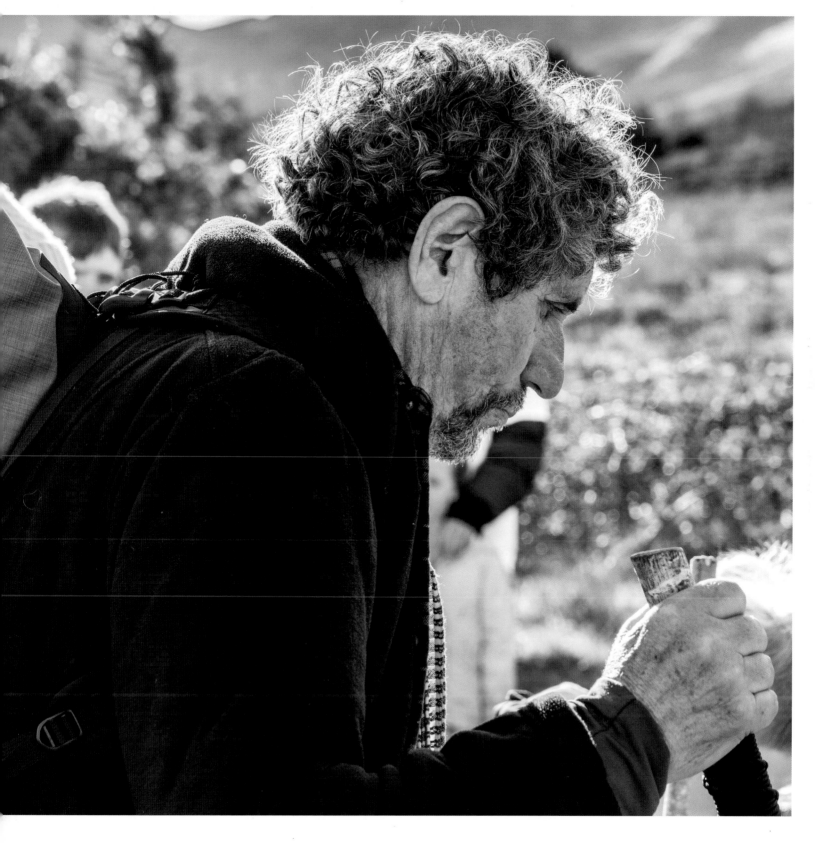

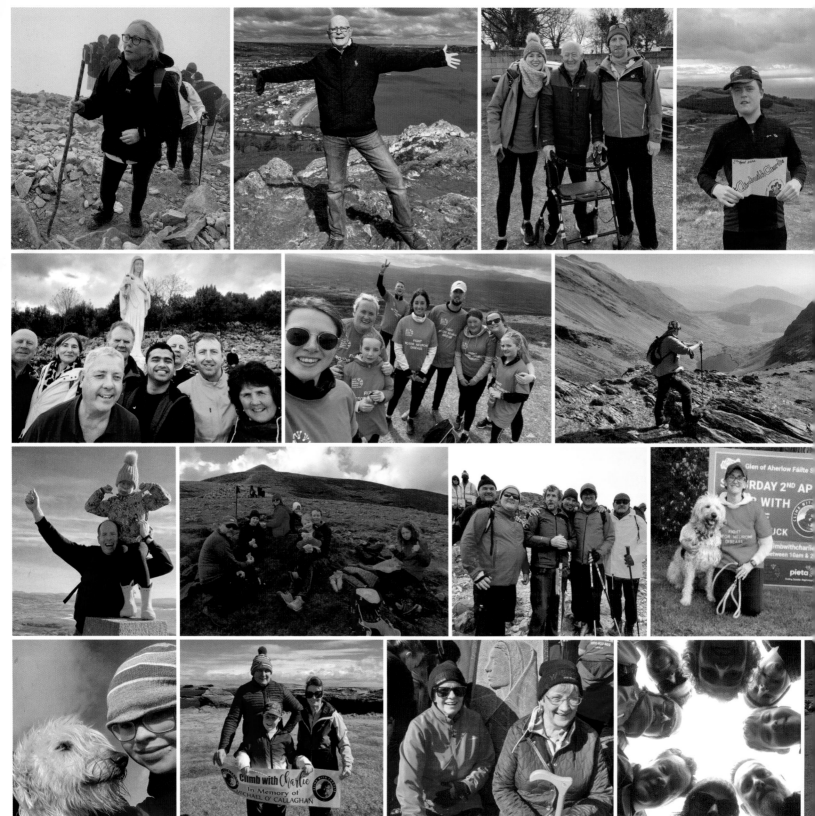

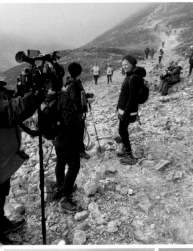
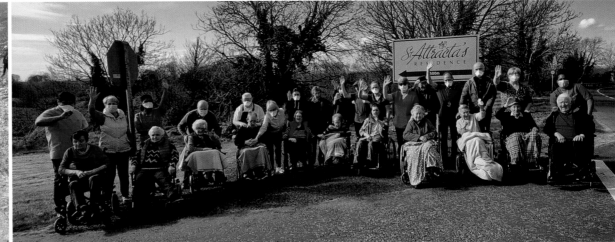
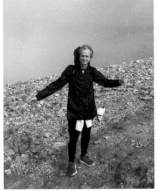
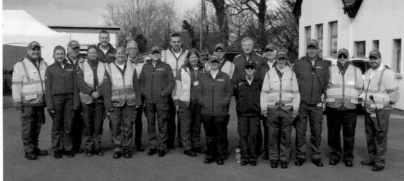
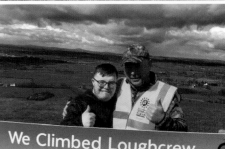

We Climbed Loughcrew
For "Climb With Charlie"

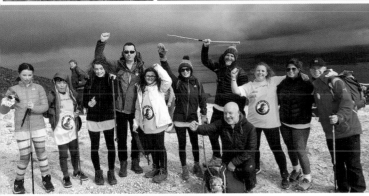
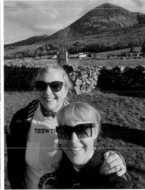
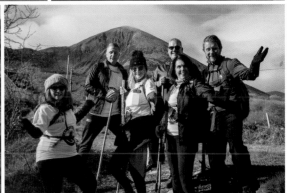
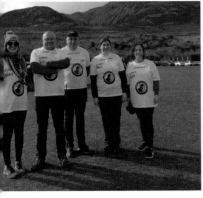
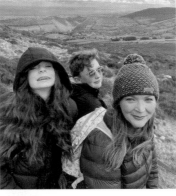
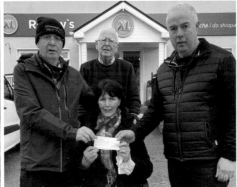
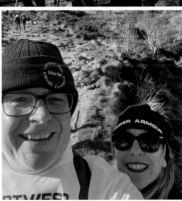

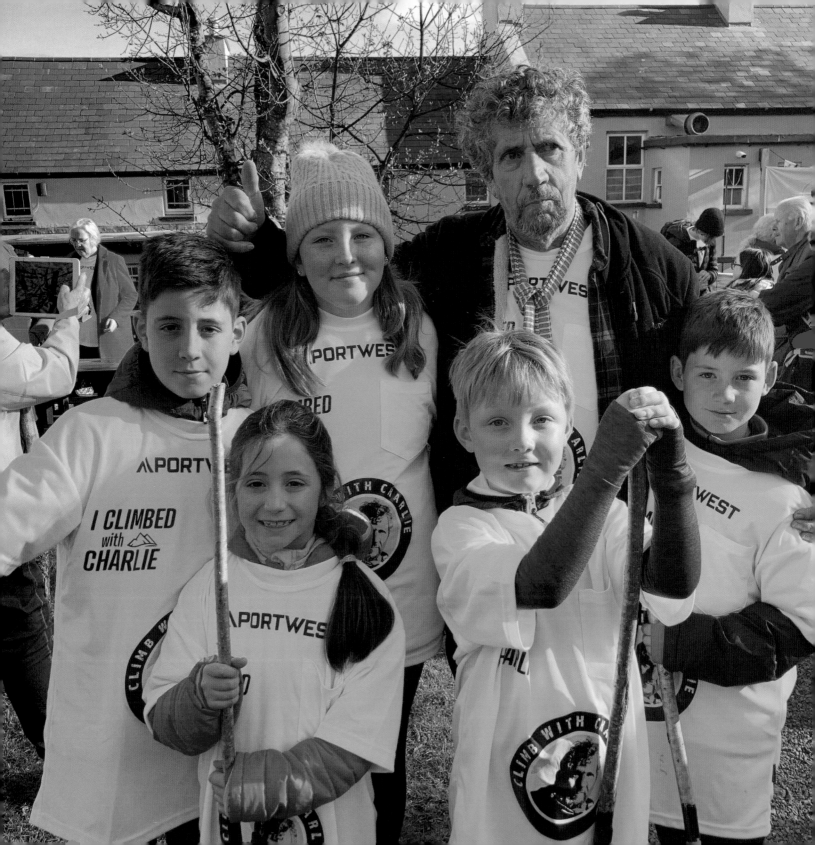

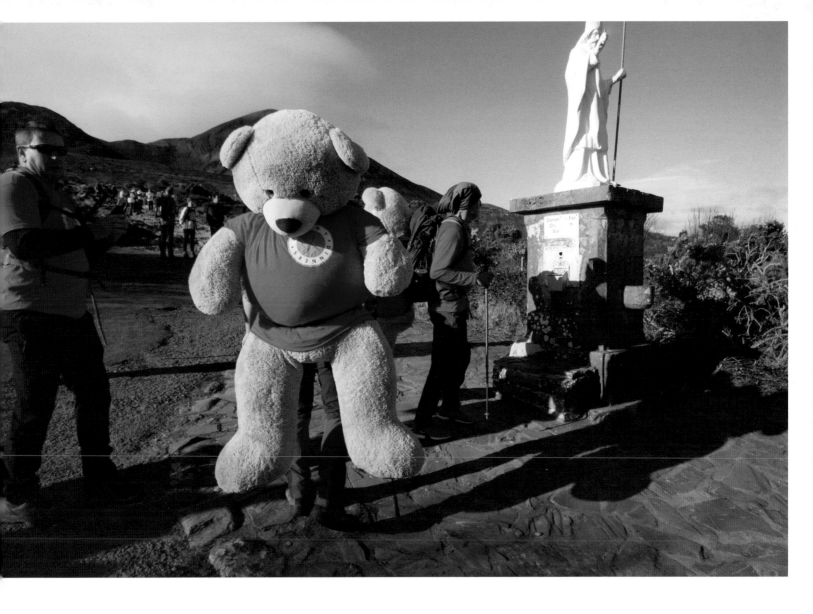

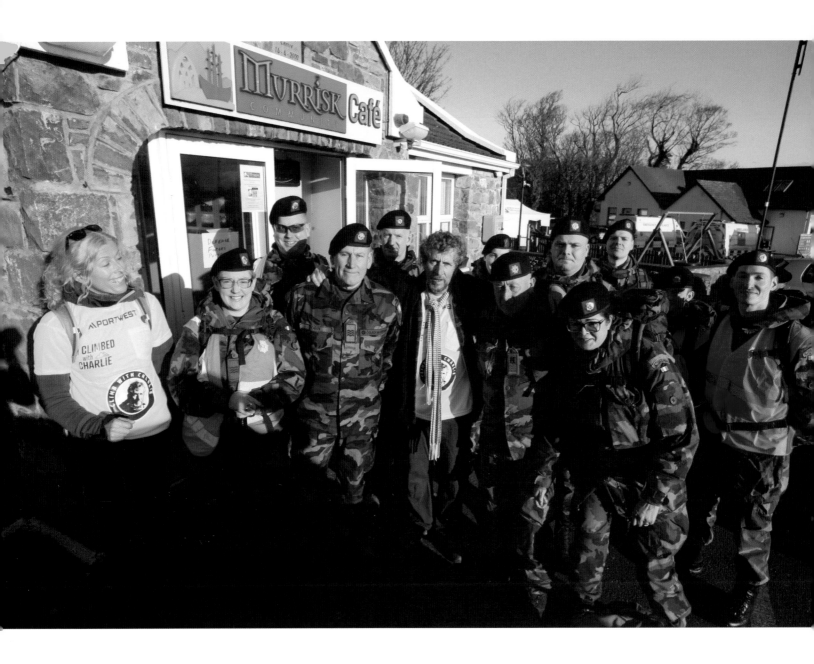

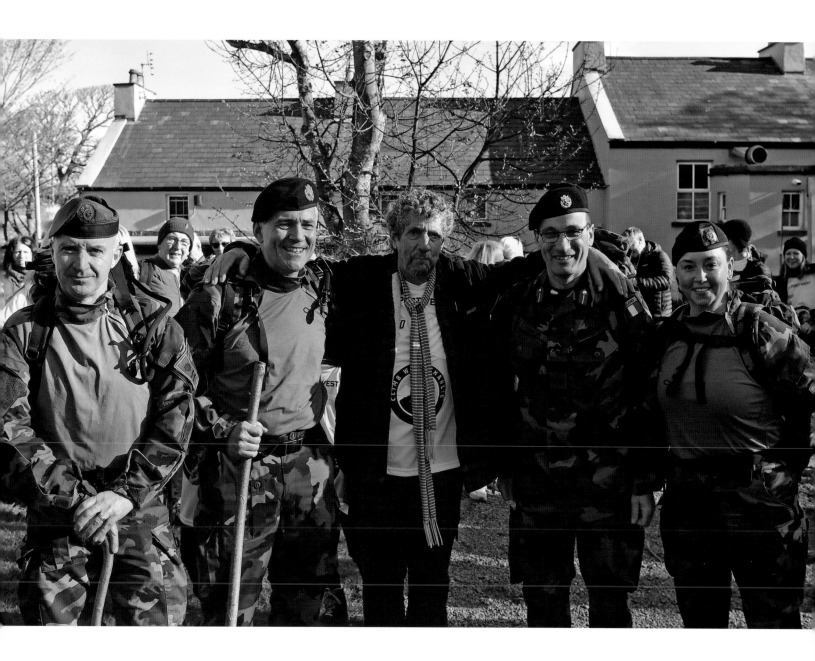

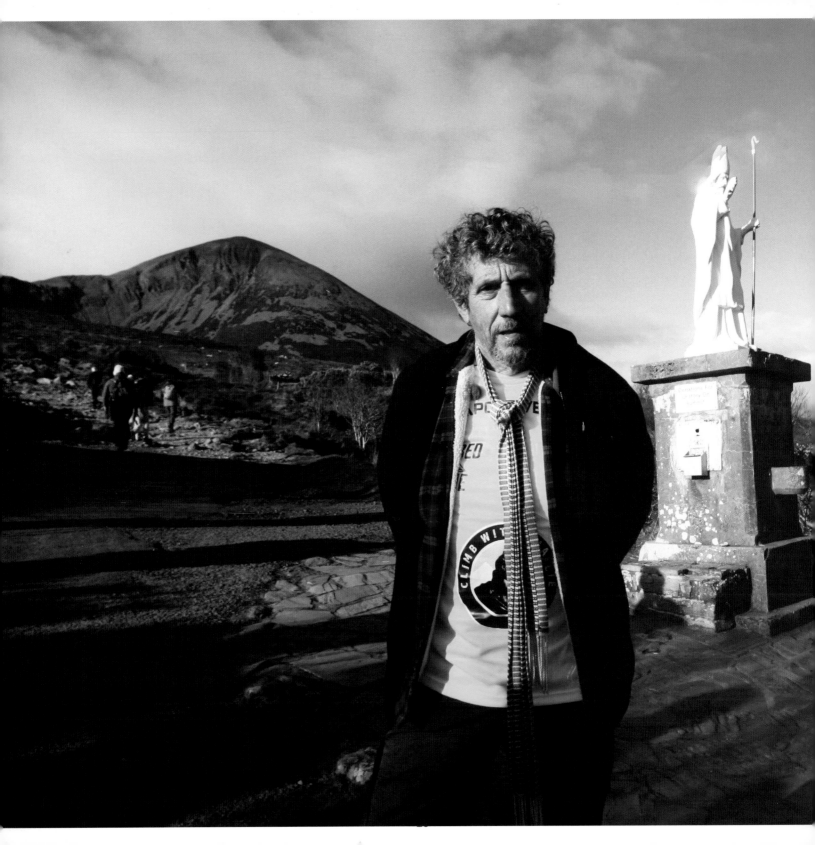

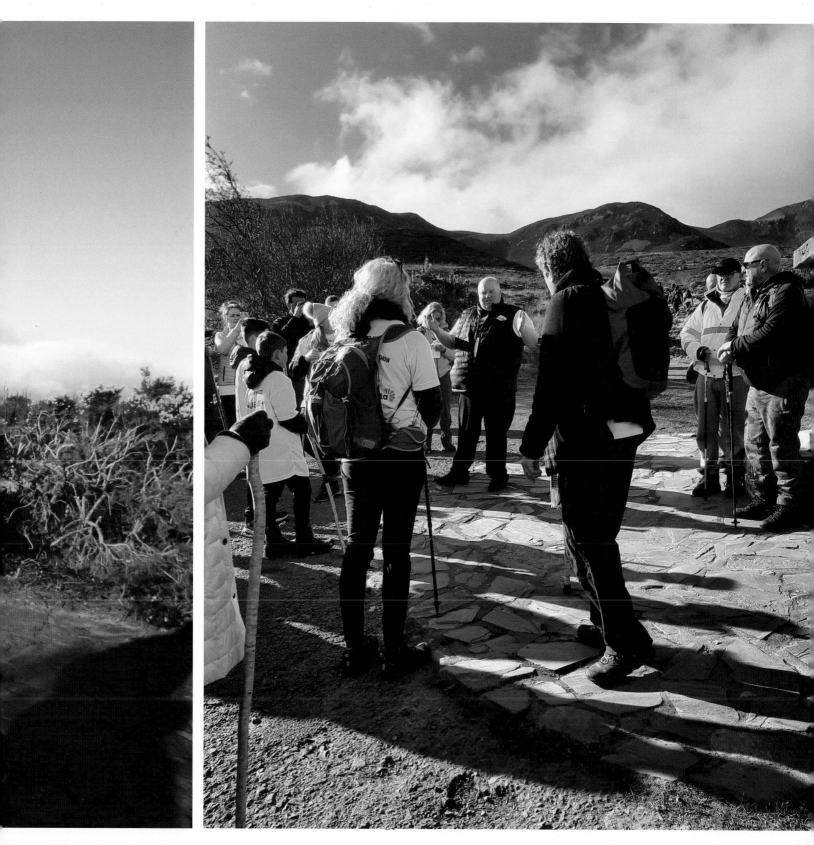

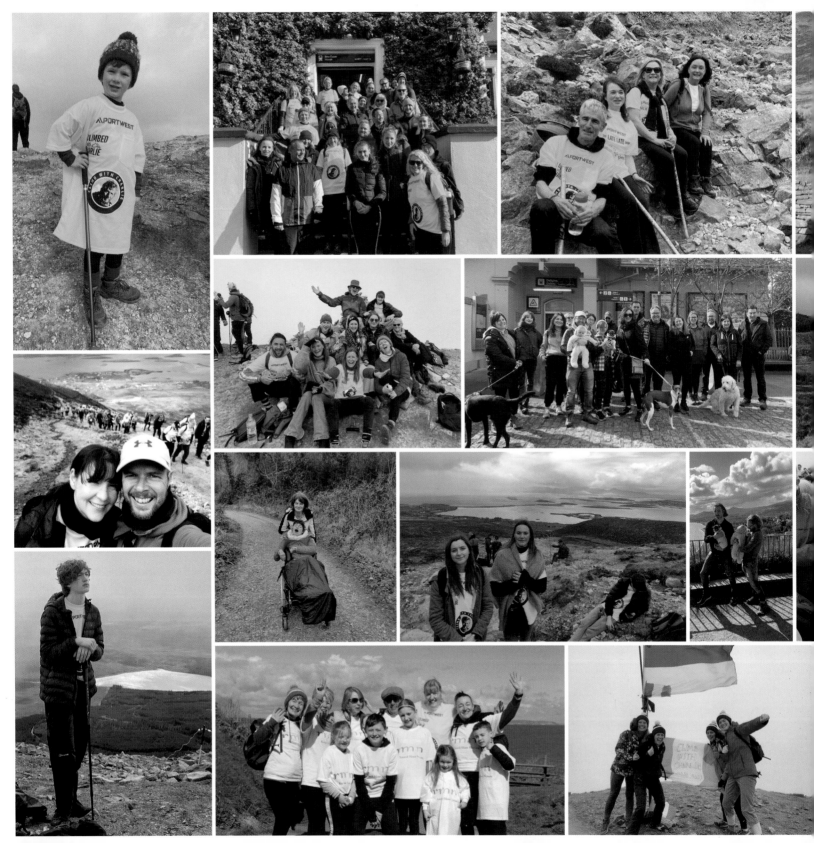

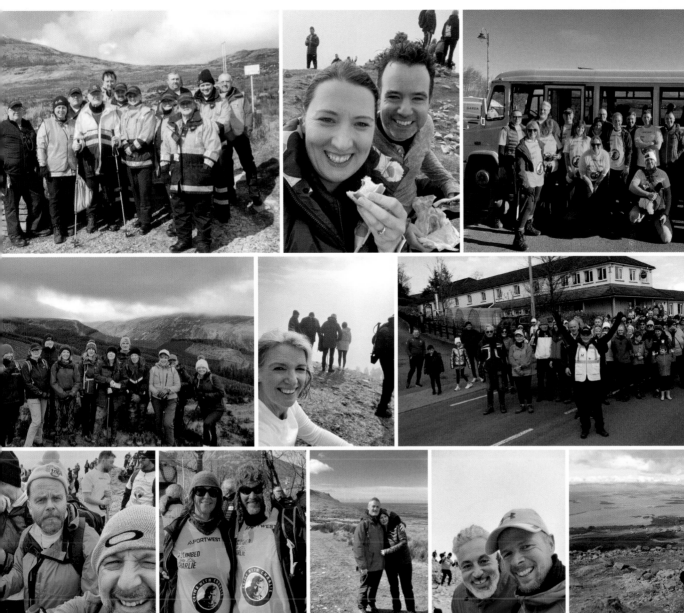
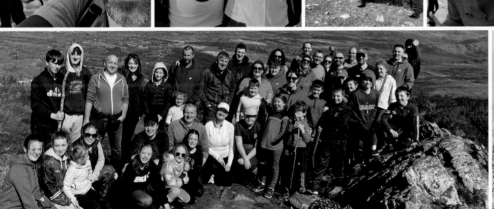
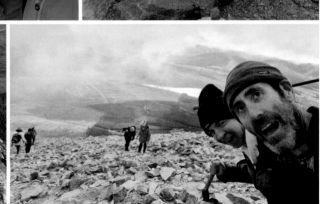

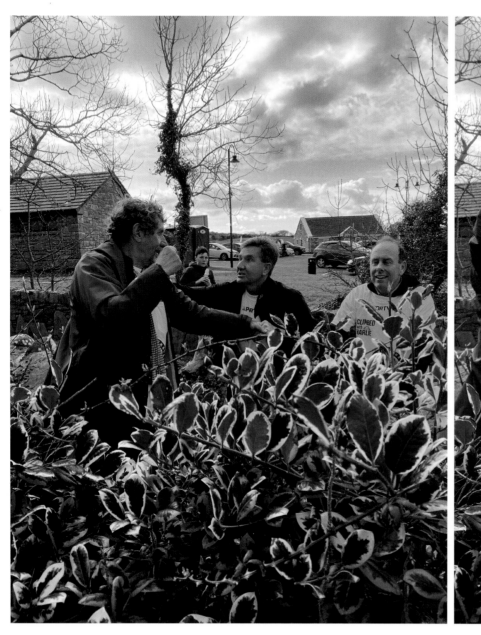
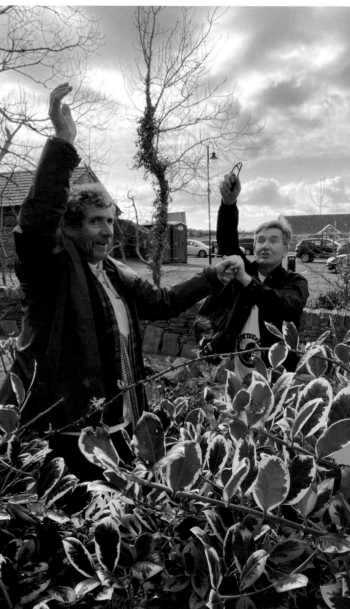

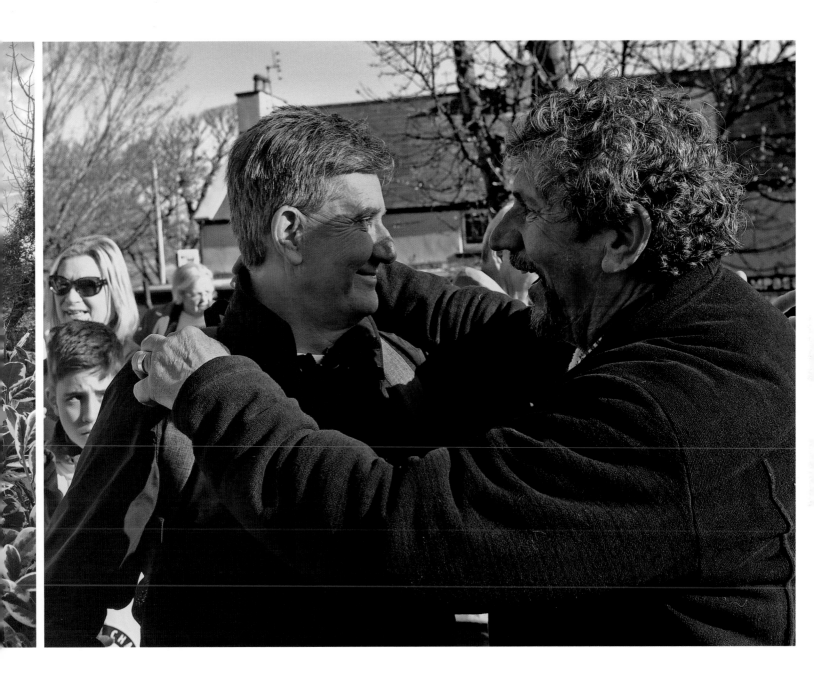

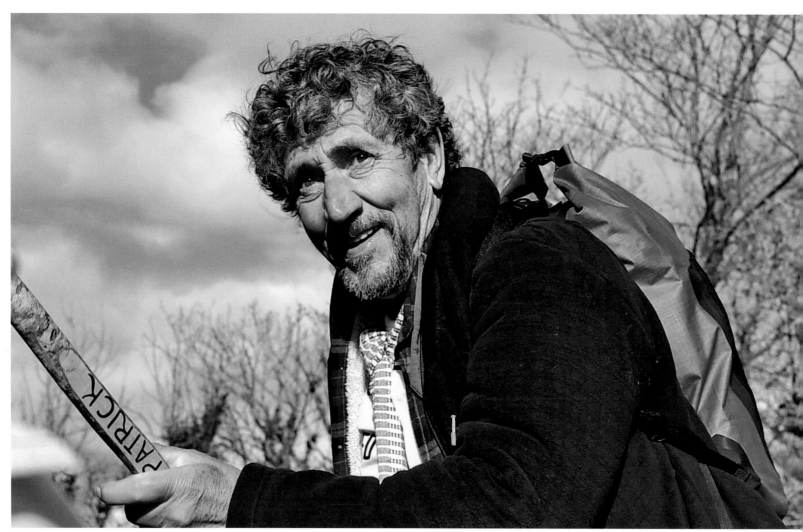

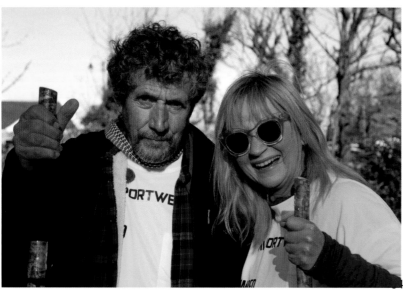

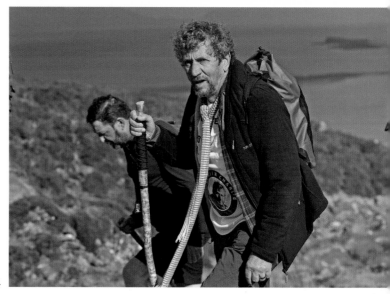

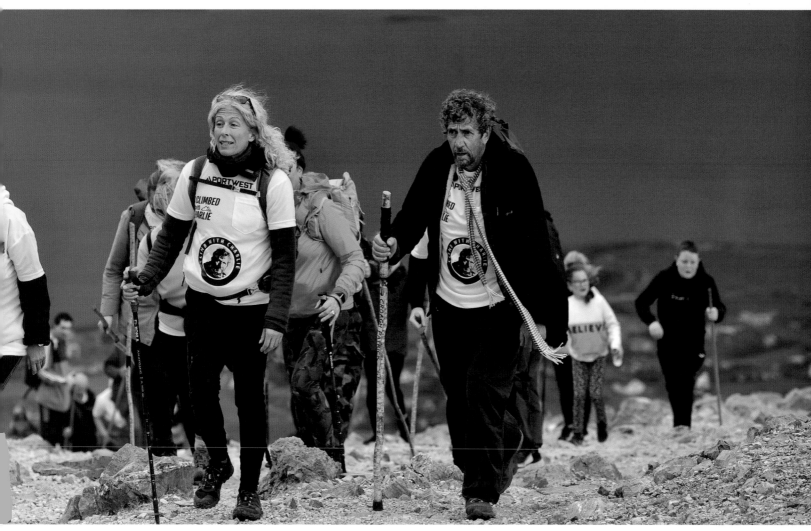
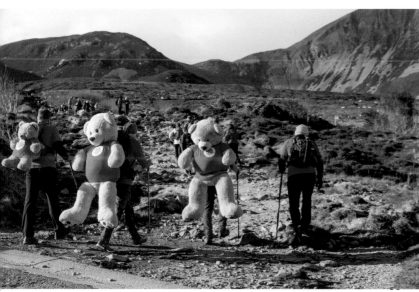
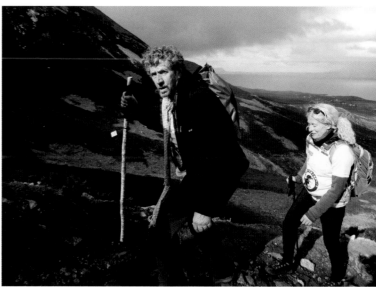

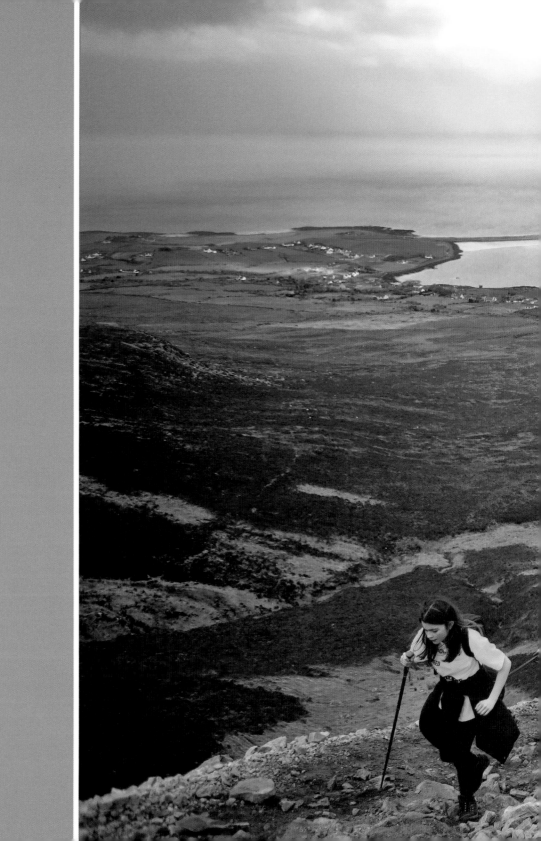

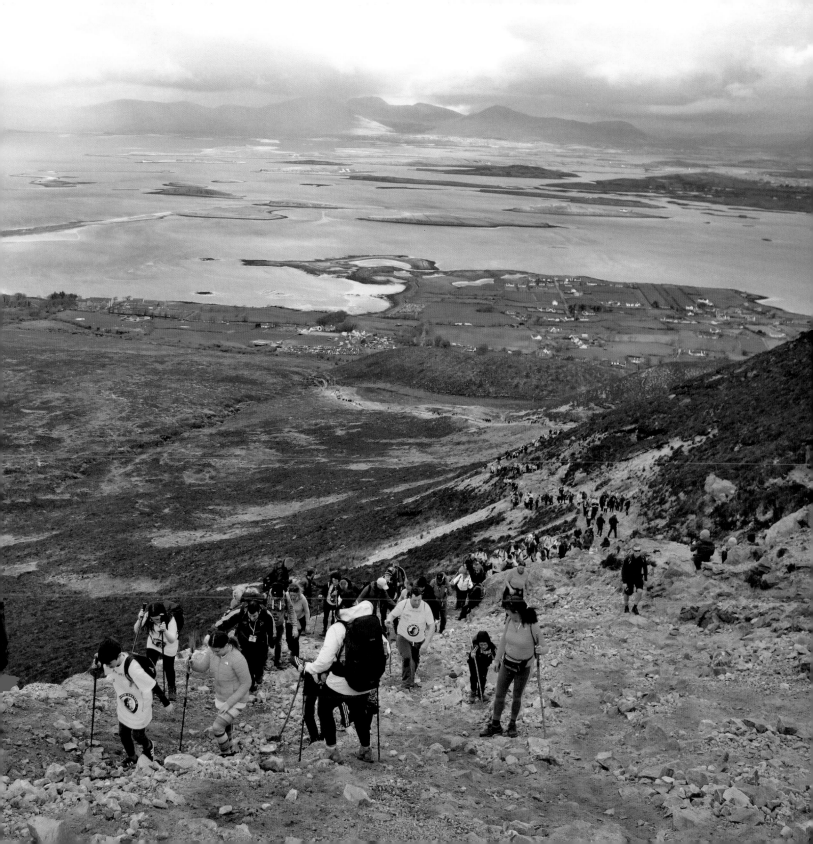

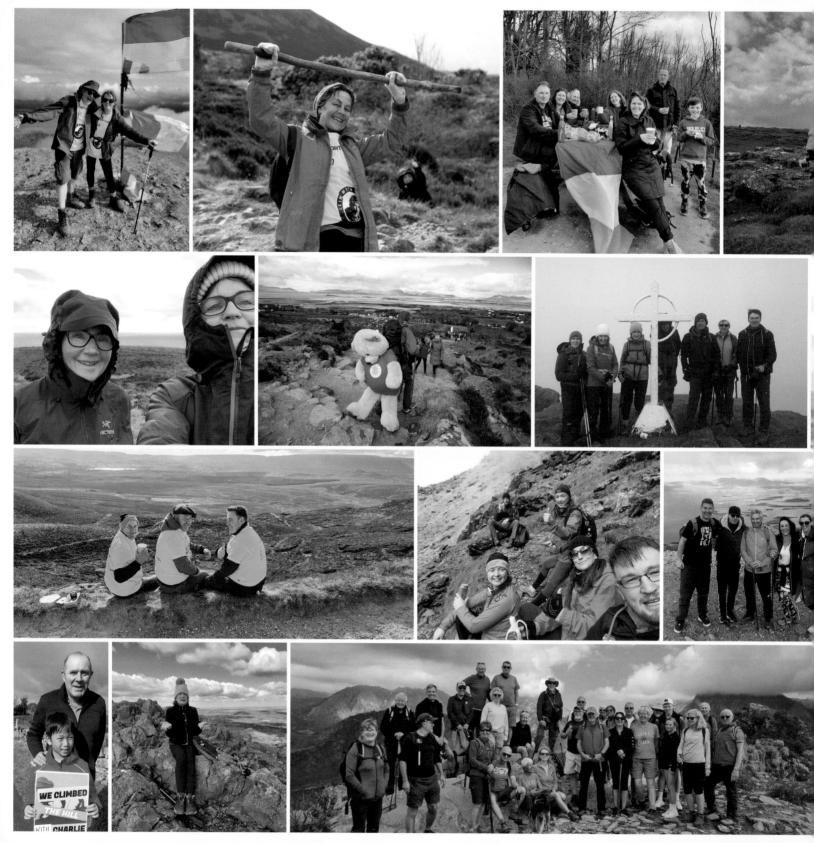

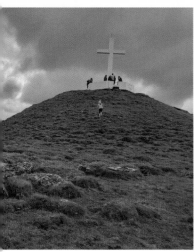
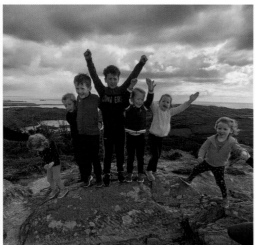
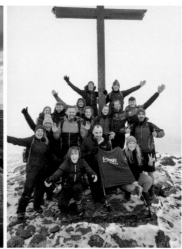
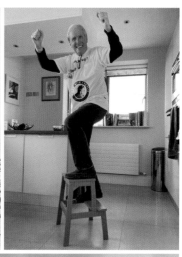

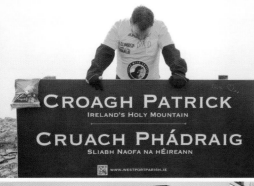
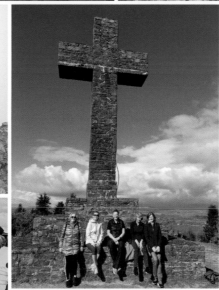
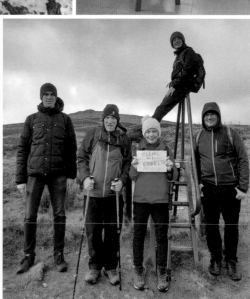

CROAGH PATRICK
IRELAND'S HOLY MOUNTAIN

CRUACH PHÁDRAIG
SLIABH NAOFA NA HÉIREANN

WWW.WESTPORTPARISH.IE

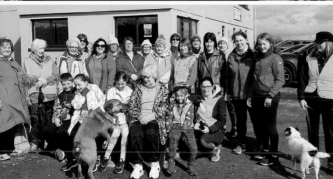
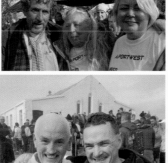

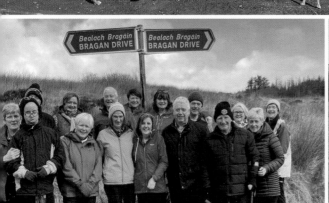
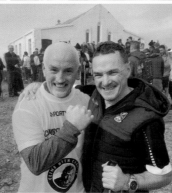
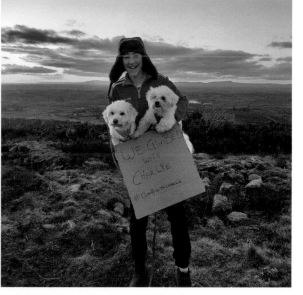

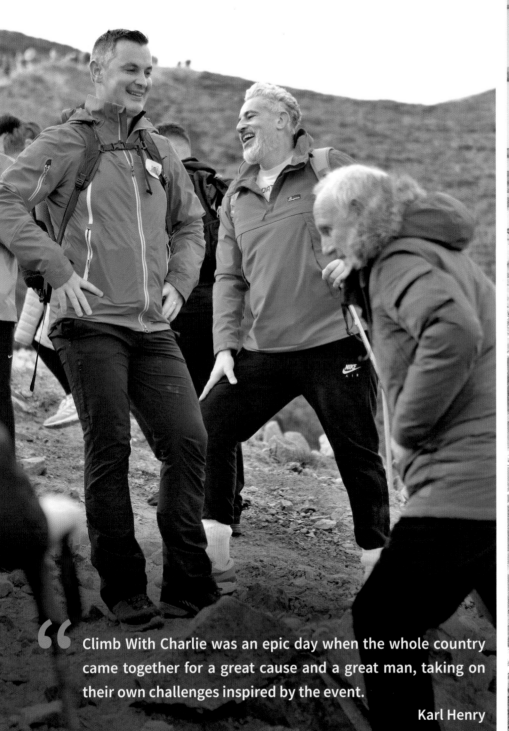

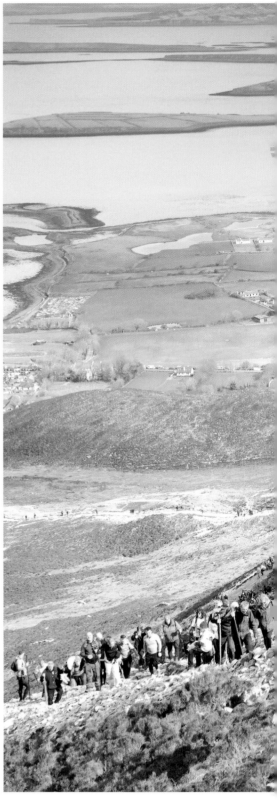

> "Climb With Charlie was an epic day when the whole country came together for a great cause and a great man, taking on their own challenges inspired by the event.
>
> Karl Henry

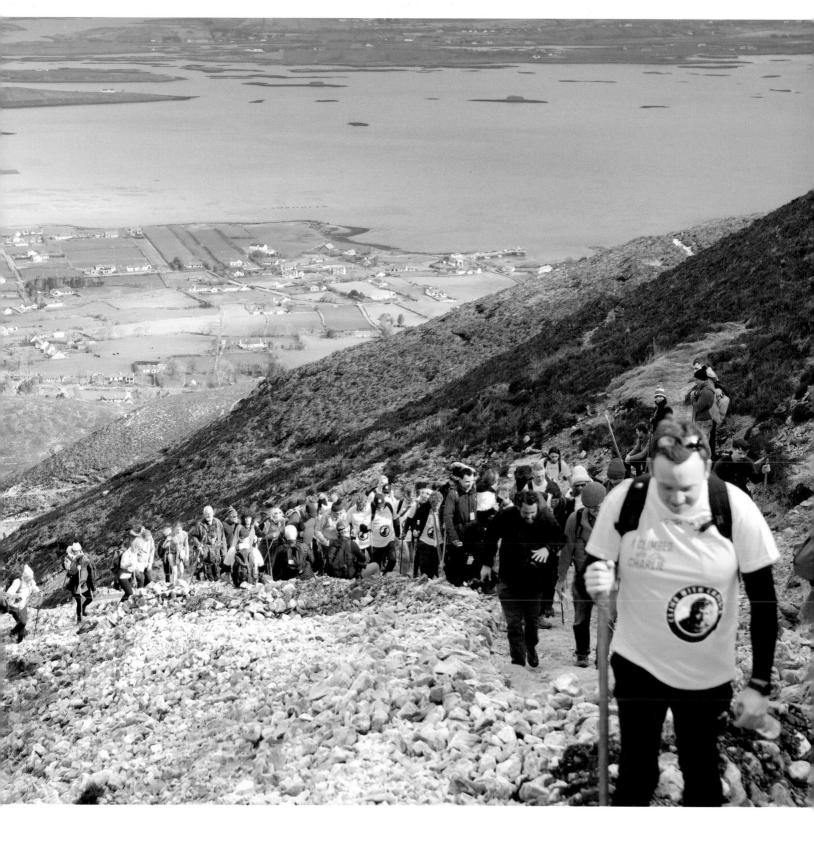

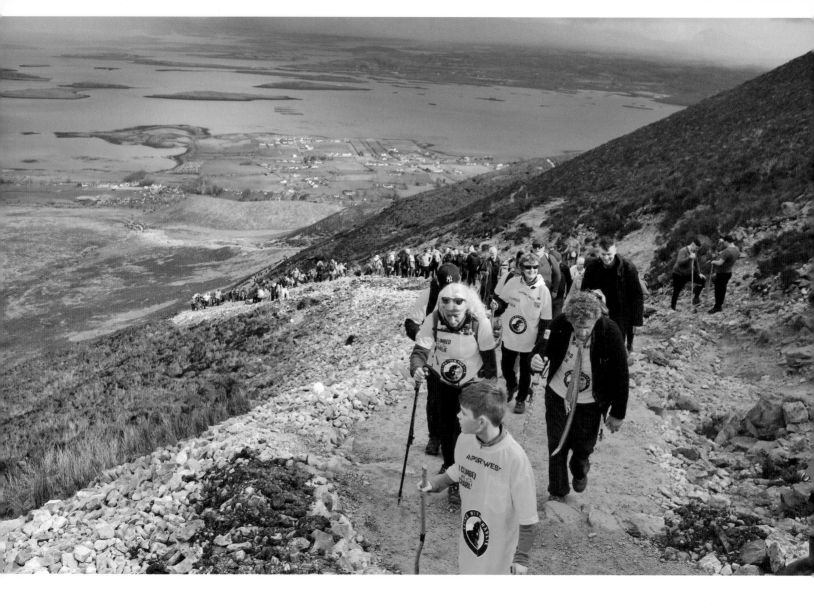

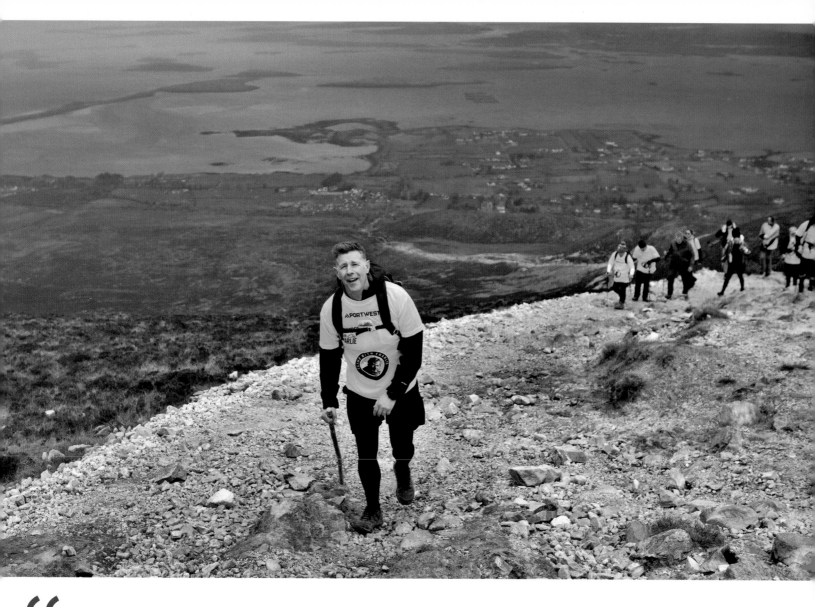

" It was an incredible honour to have been asked to accompany Charlie up Croagh Patrick that April morning. It felt like Charlie, Claire and their family were leading the entire country up the mountain. Charlie was inspirational, as I knew he would be, but what I wasn't prepared for was the togetherness of everyone who climbed, their patience with, help for and encouragement to each other; everyone was climbing in solidarity. There was laughter, kindness, tears and friendship. Charlie set out to open our eyes to and embrace those around us who are suffering in silence, to show them we care. He did that and I feel privileged to have witnessed it. It was a day I will never forget.

Dermot Bannon

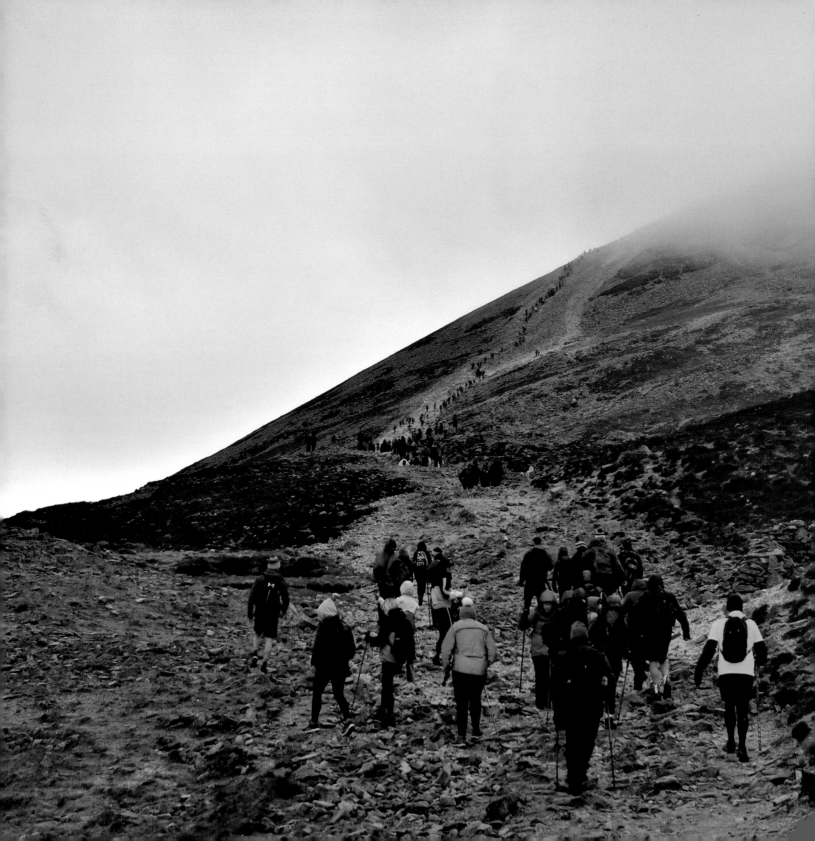

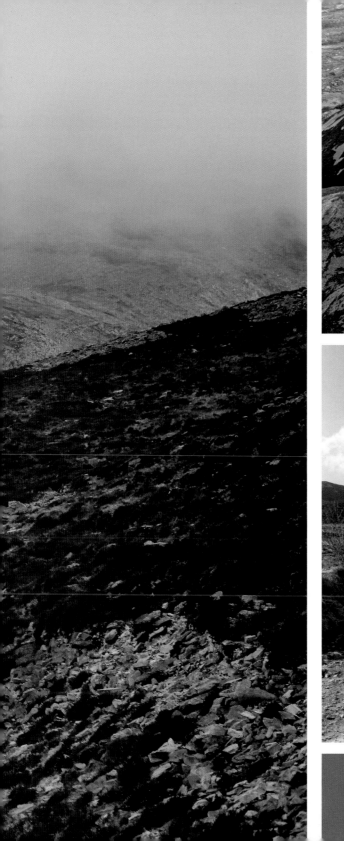
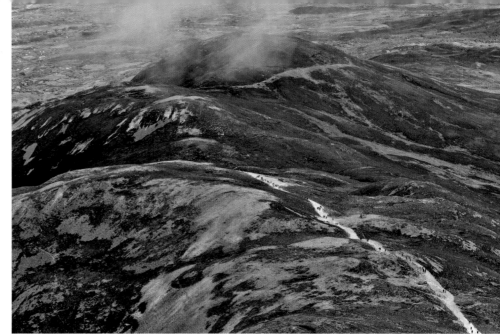
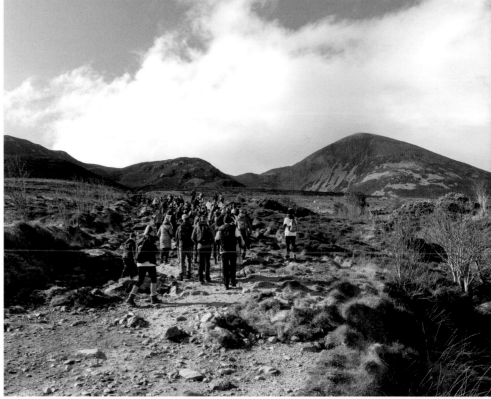

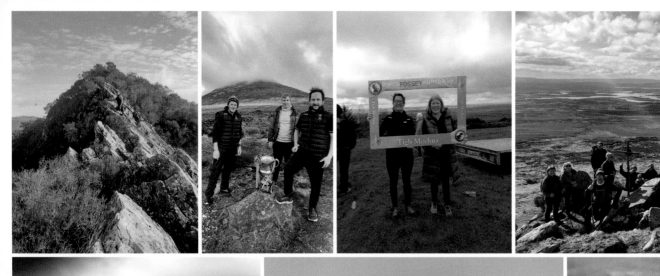
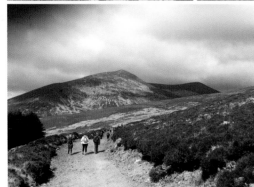
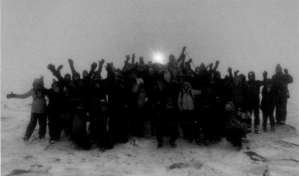
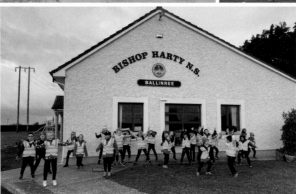
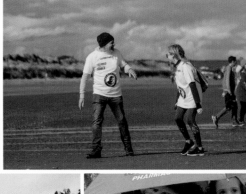
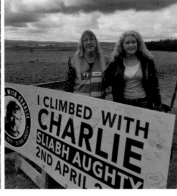
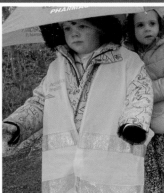
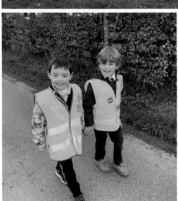
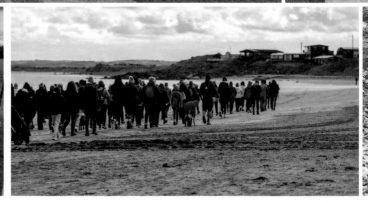

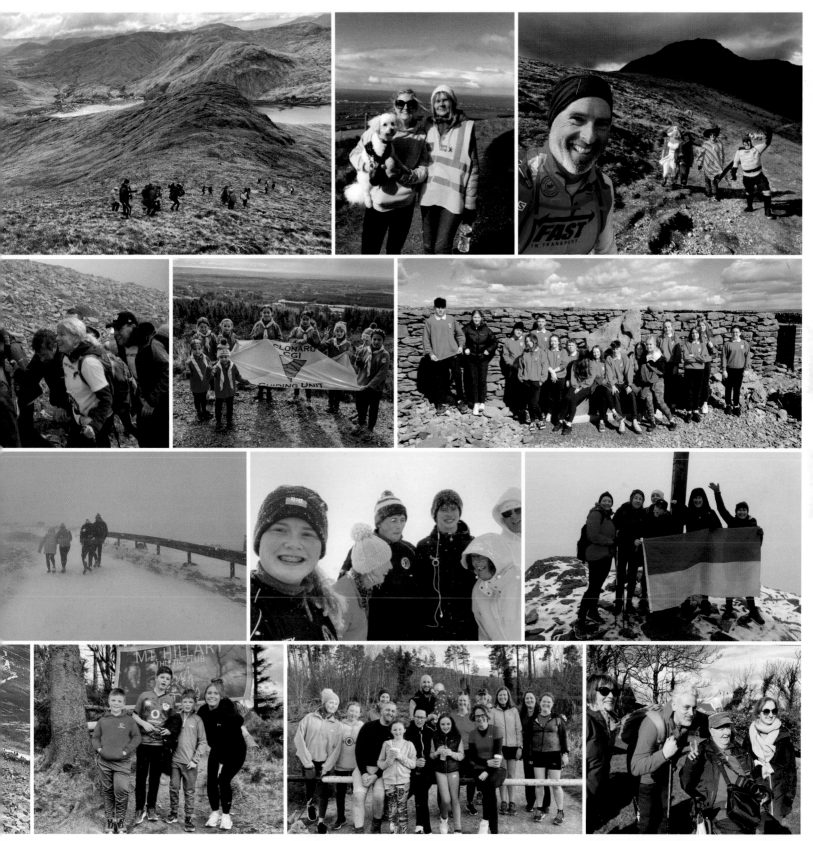

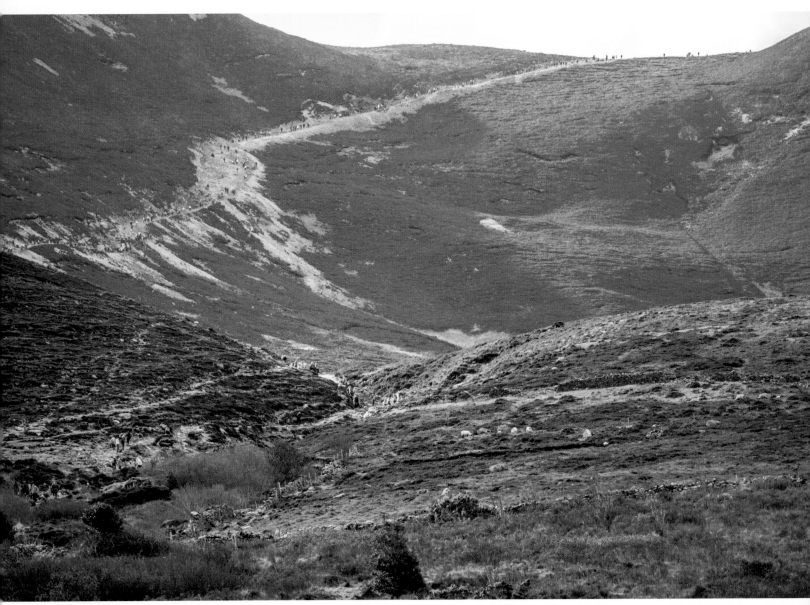

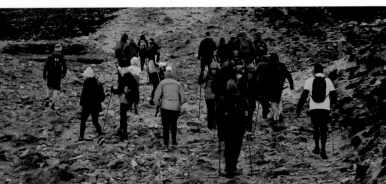

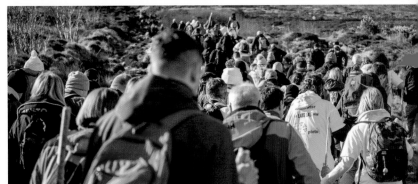

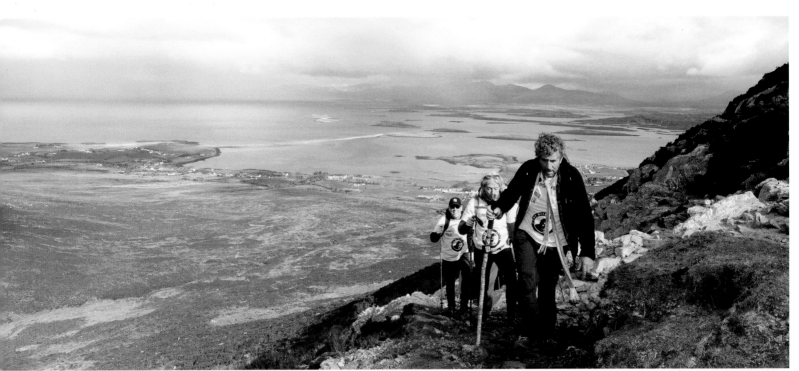

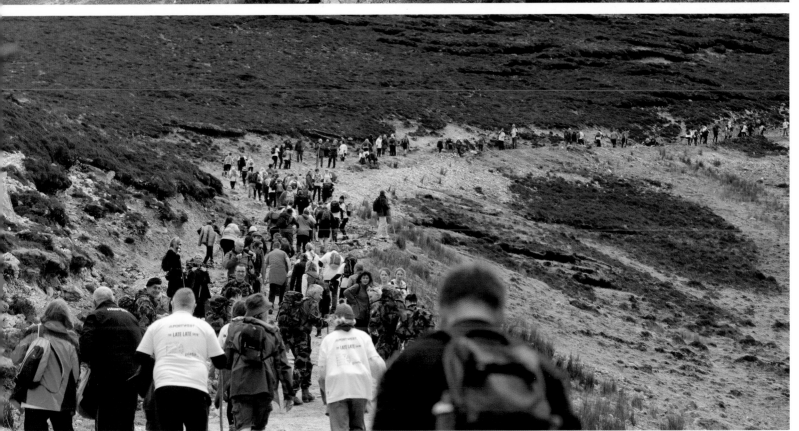

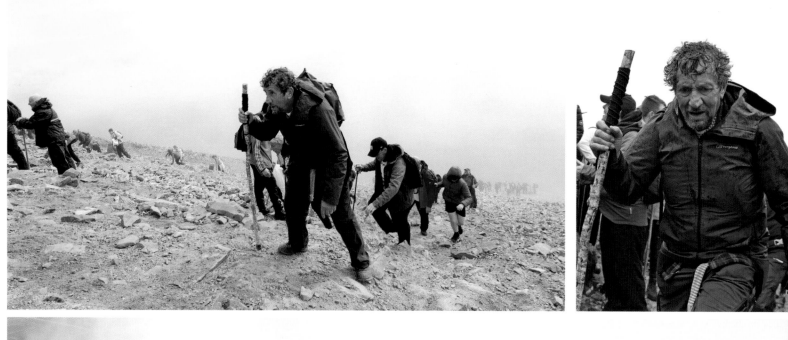
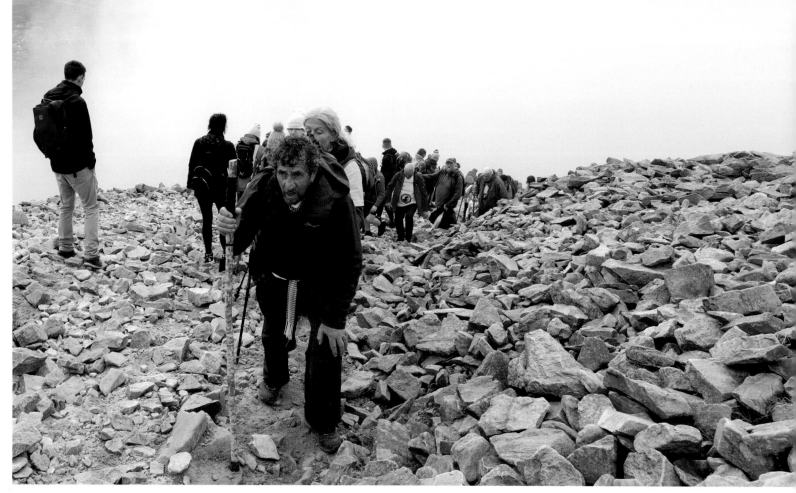

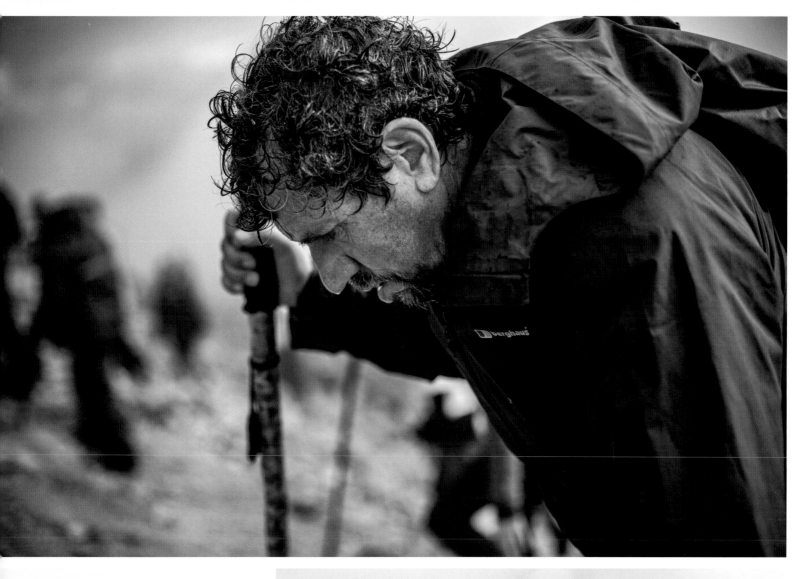

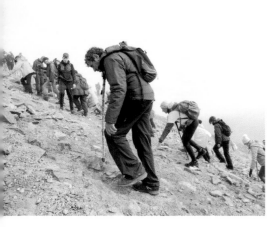

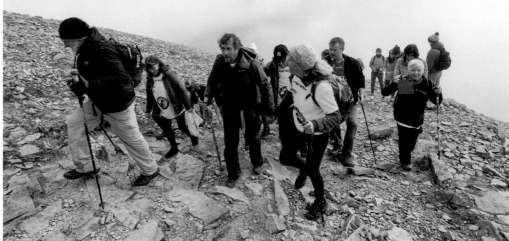

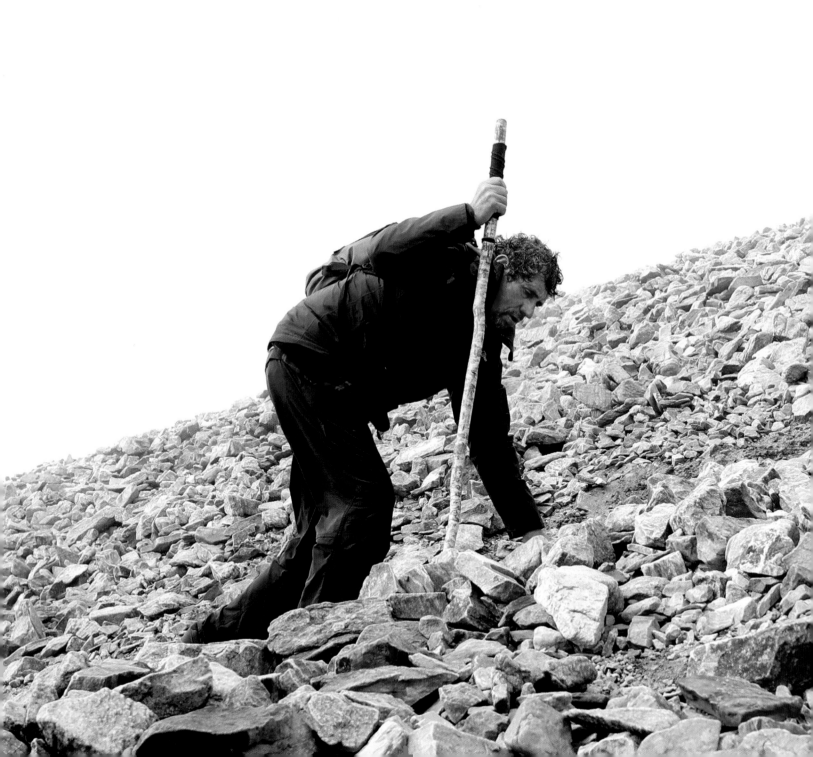

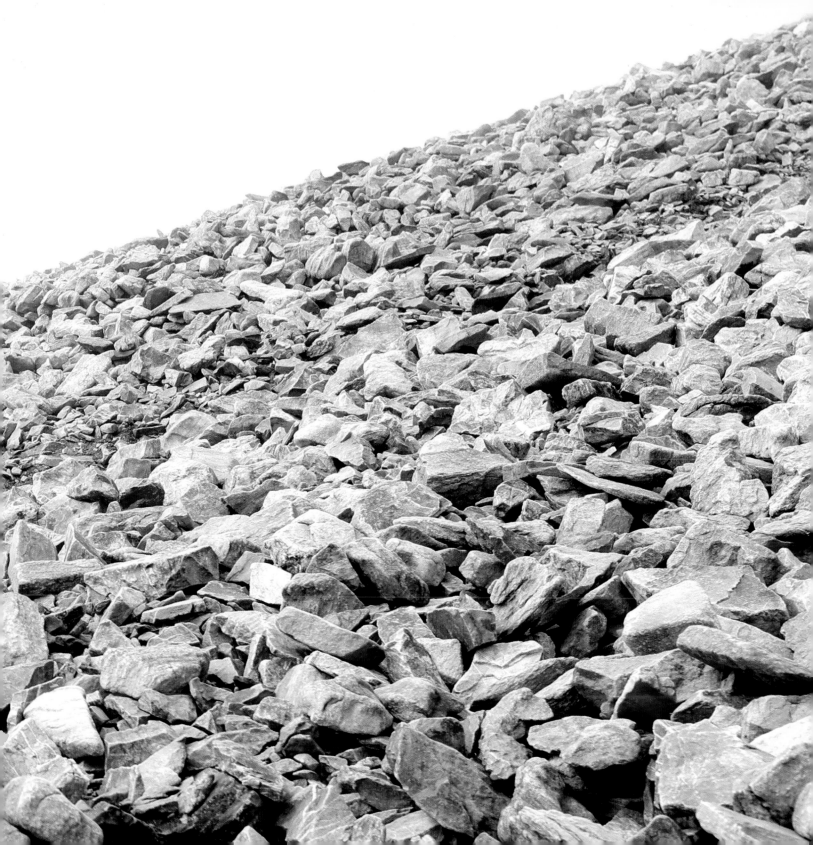

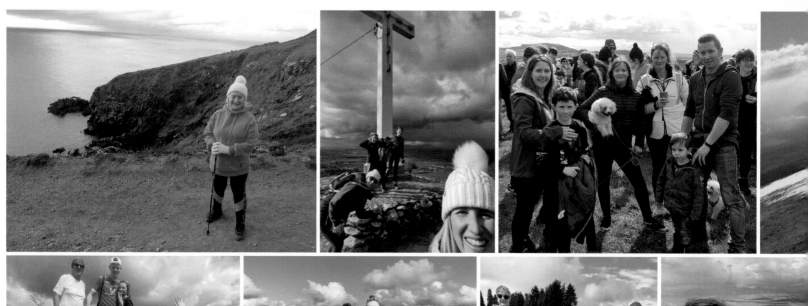
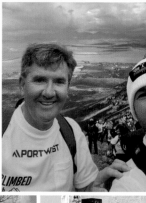
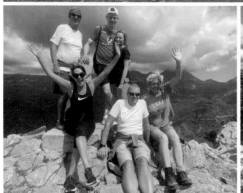
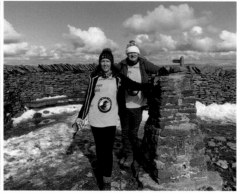
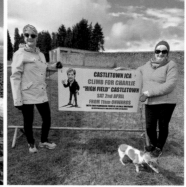
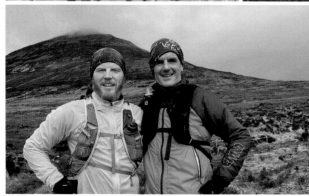
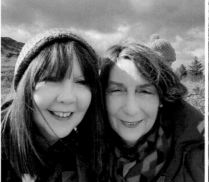
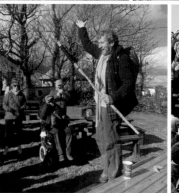
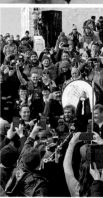
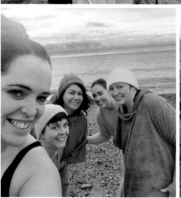
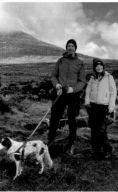
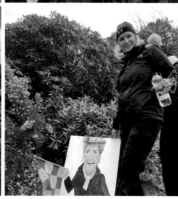
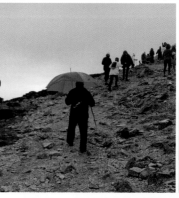
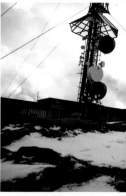

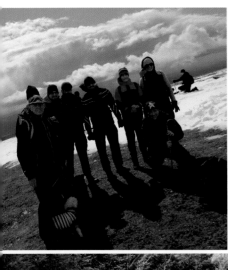
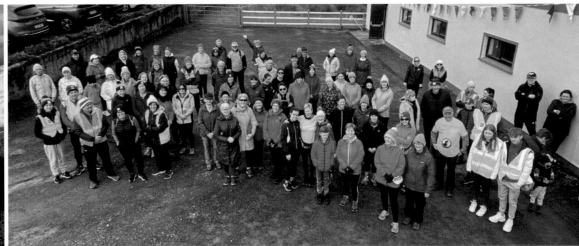
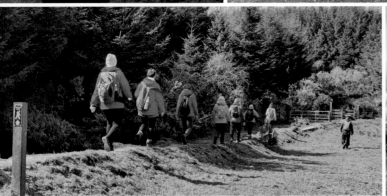
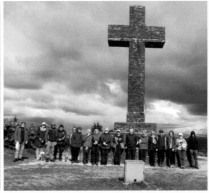
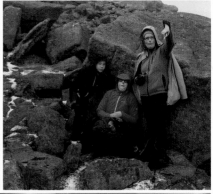
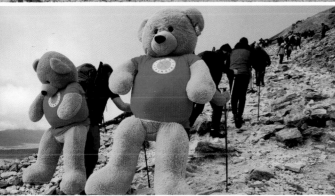
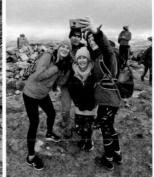
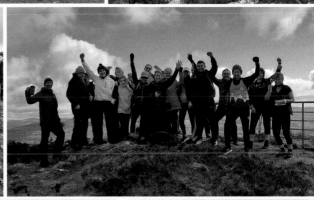
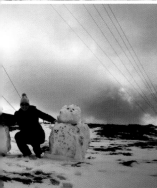
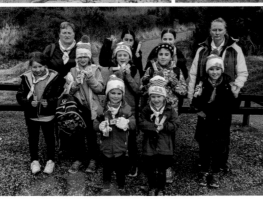
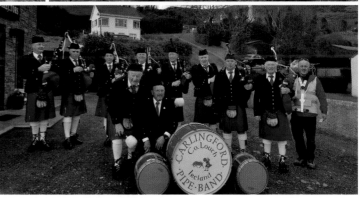

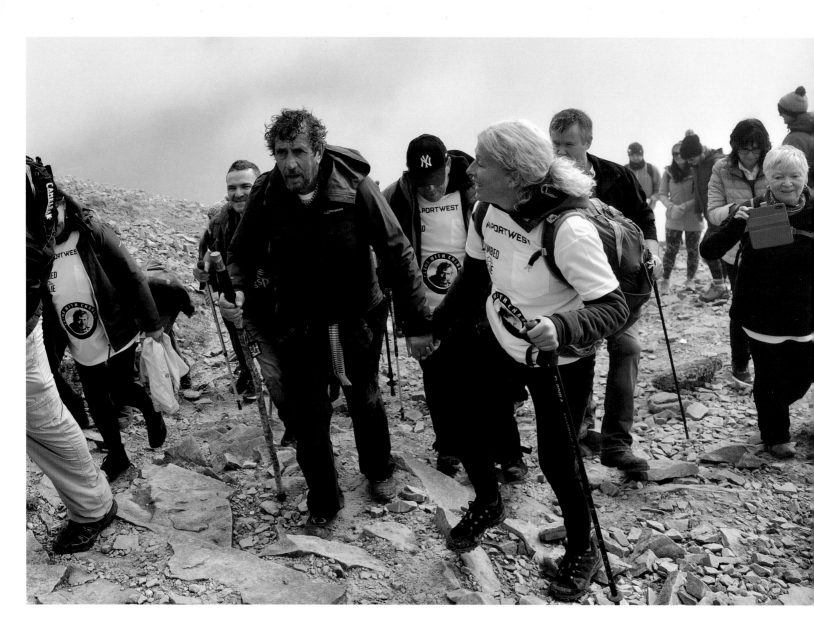

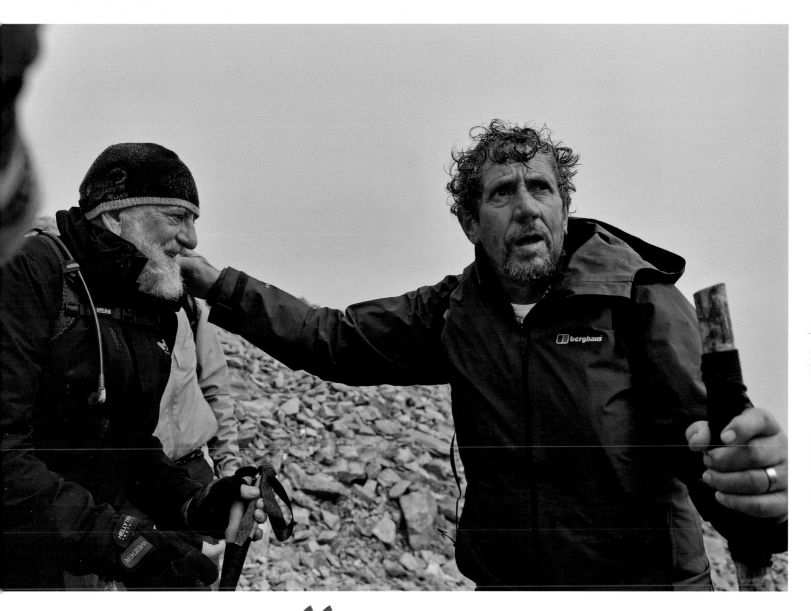

“ Charlie, it was a wonderful experience and a pleasure to climb with you and your lovely wife, Claire, to the summit of Croagh Patrick, and then to play with the Clew Bay Pipe Band at the summit, all for a great cause. A day to remember. Charlie, you're special! *Grá mór*.

Matt Molloy

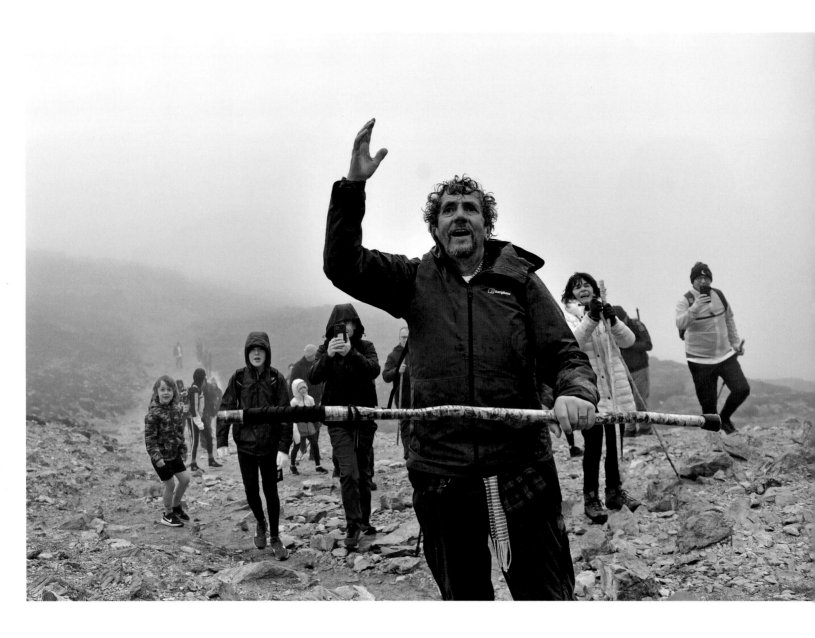

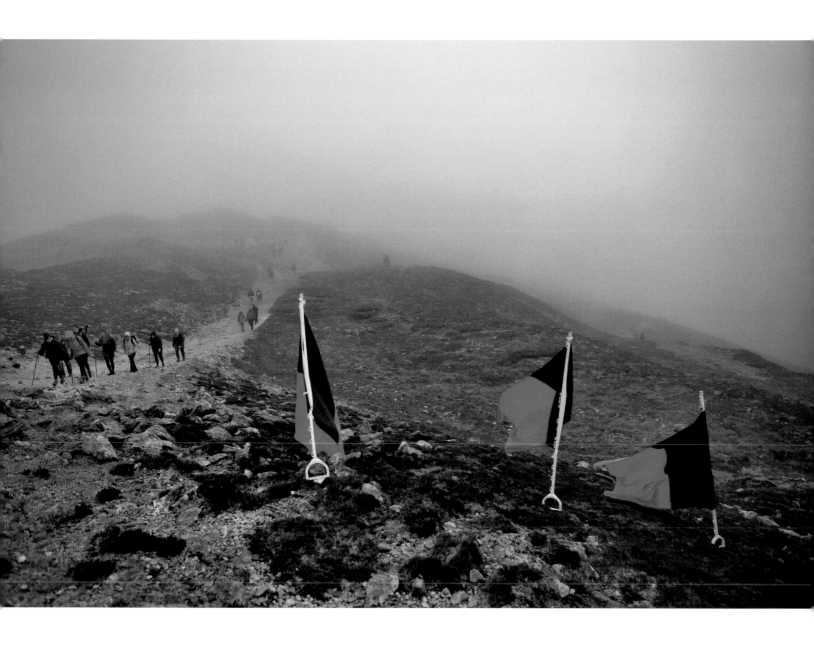

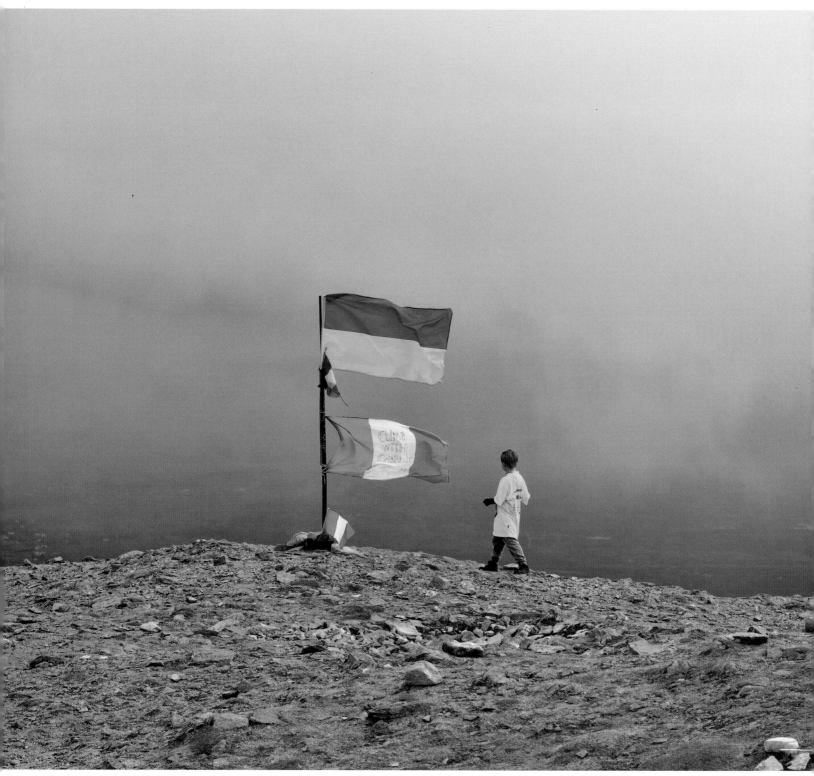

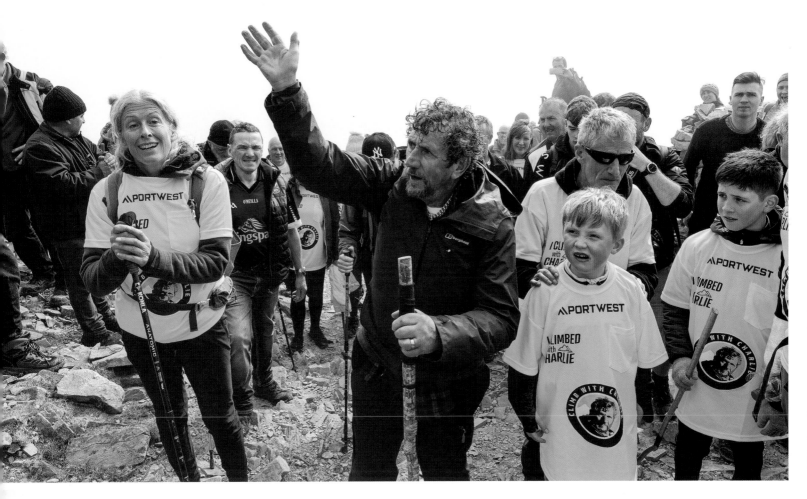

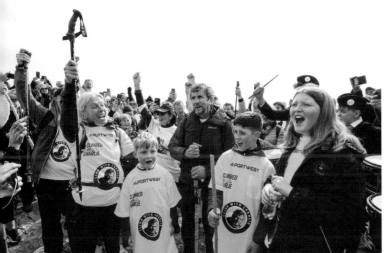

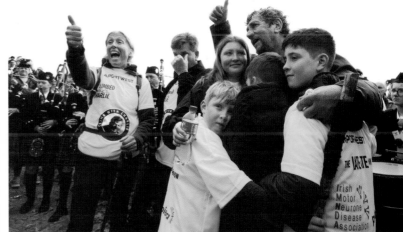

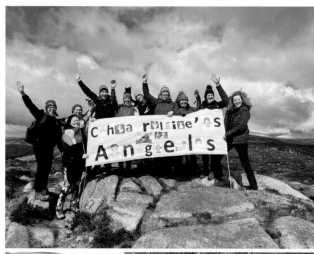
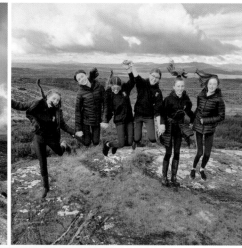
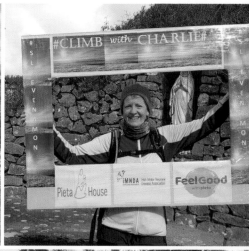
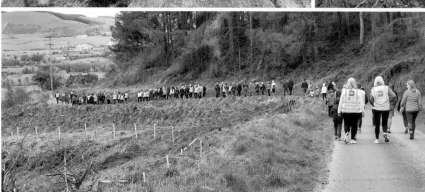
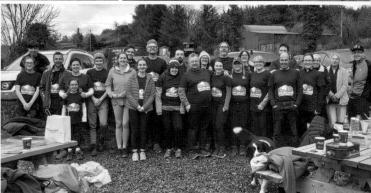
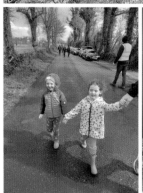
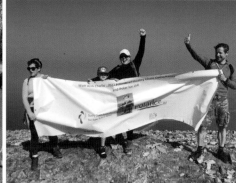
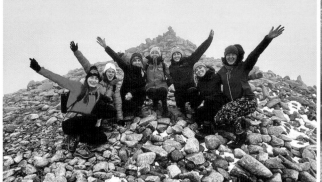
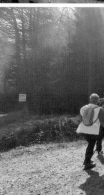
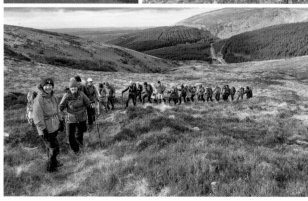
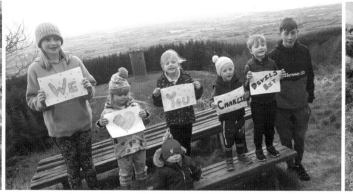
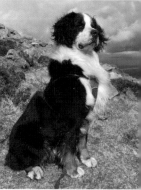

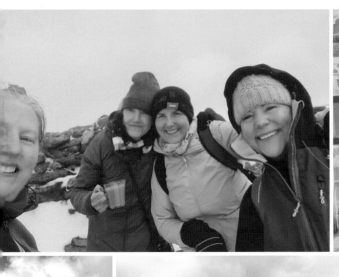
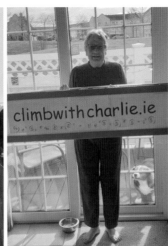
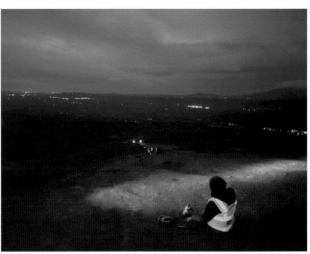
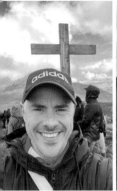
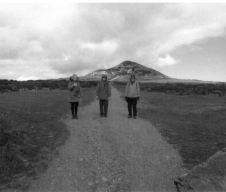
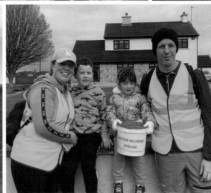
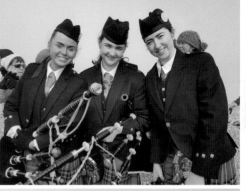
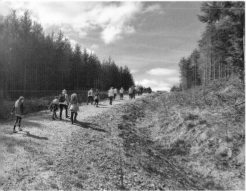
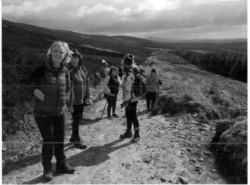
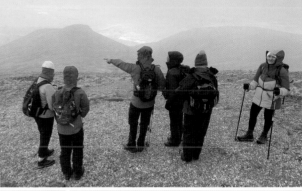
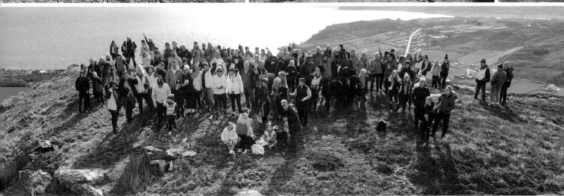
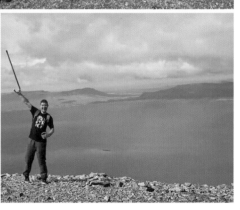

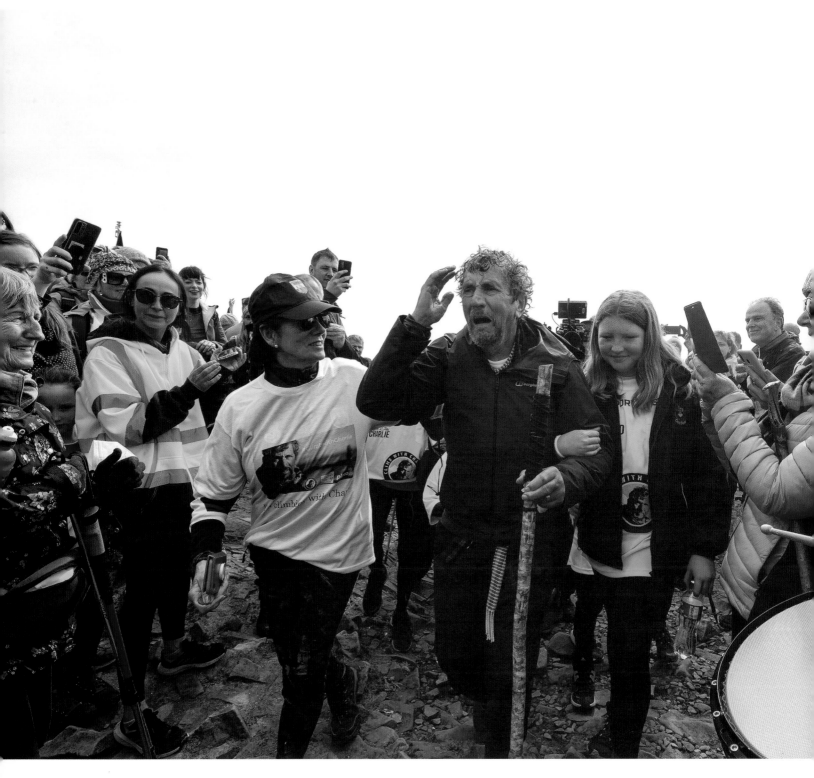

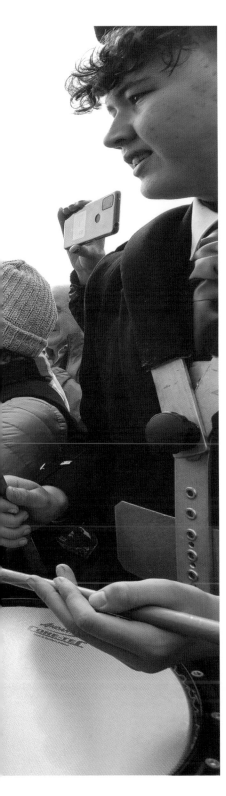
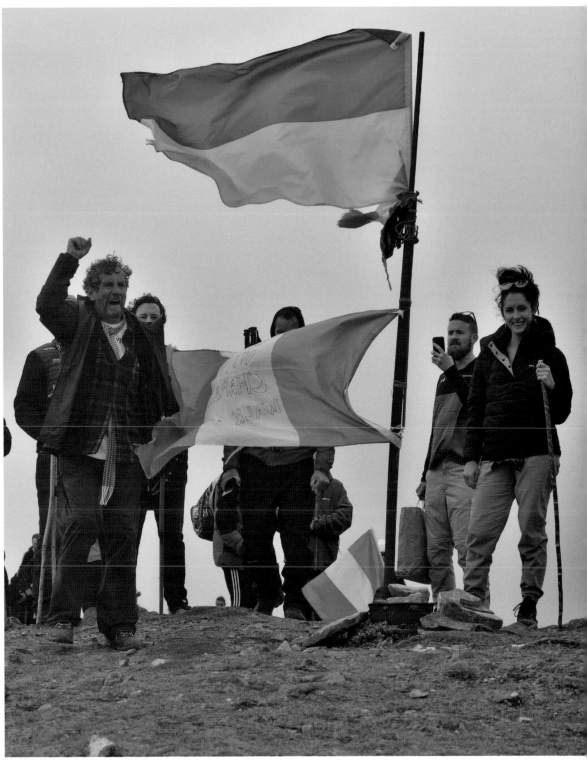

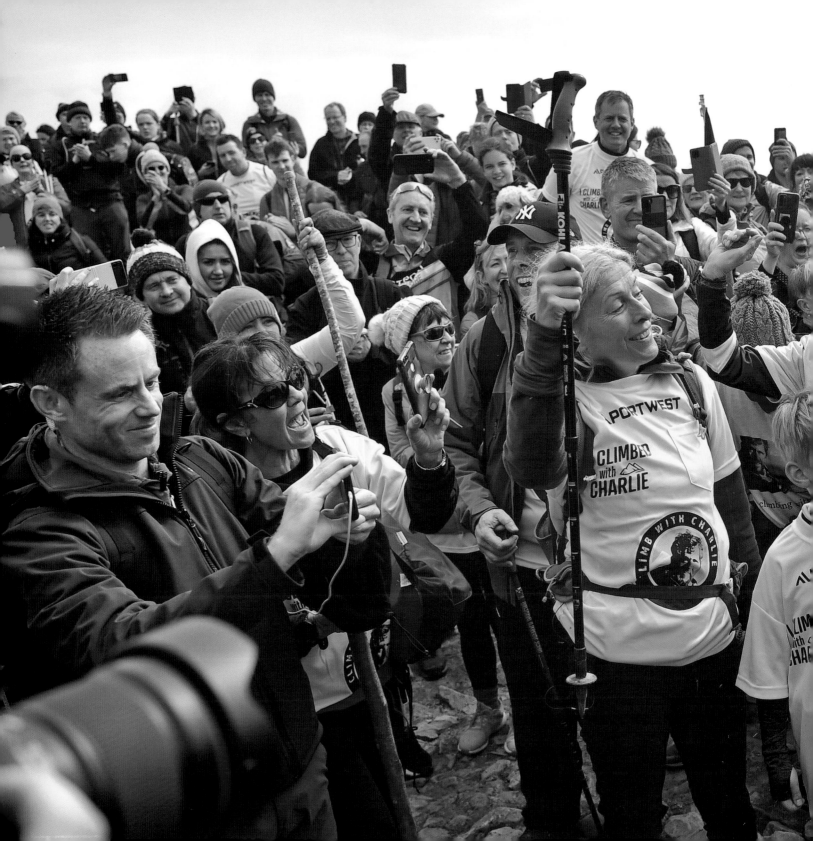

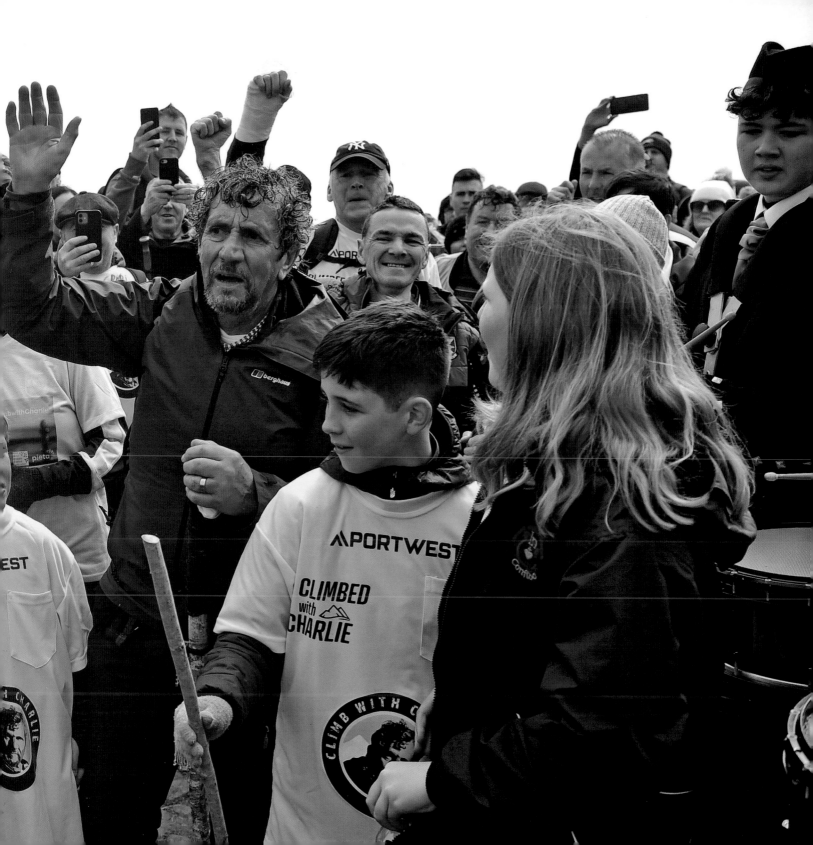

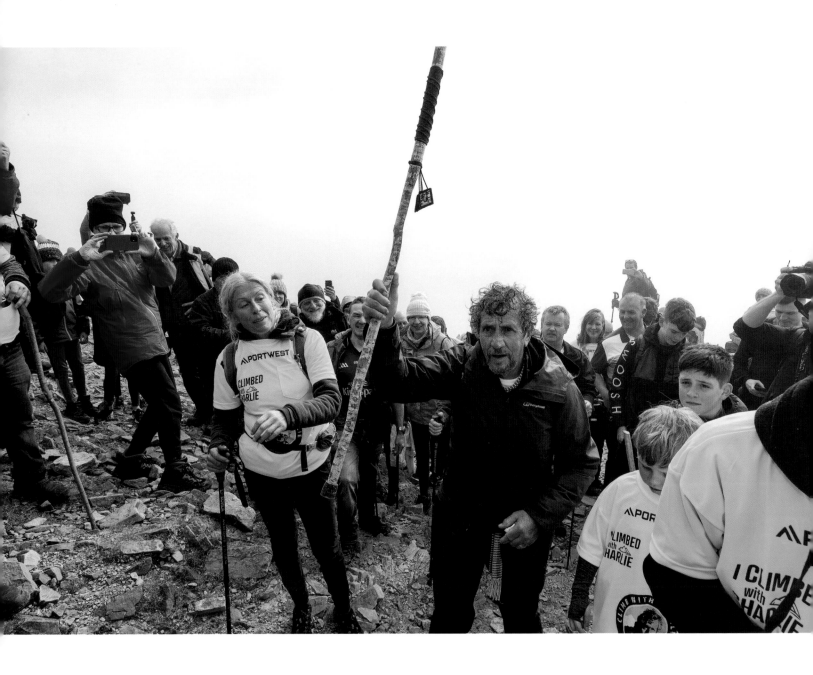

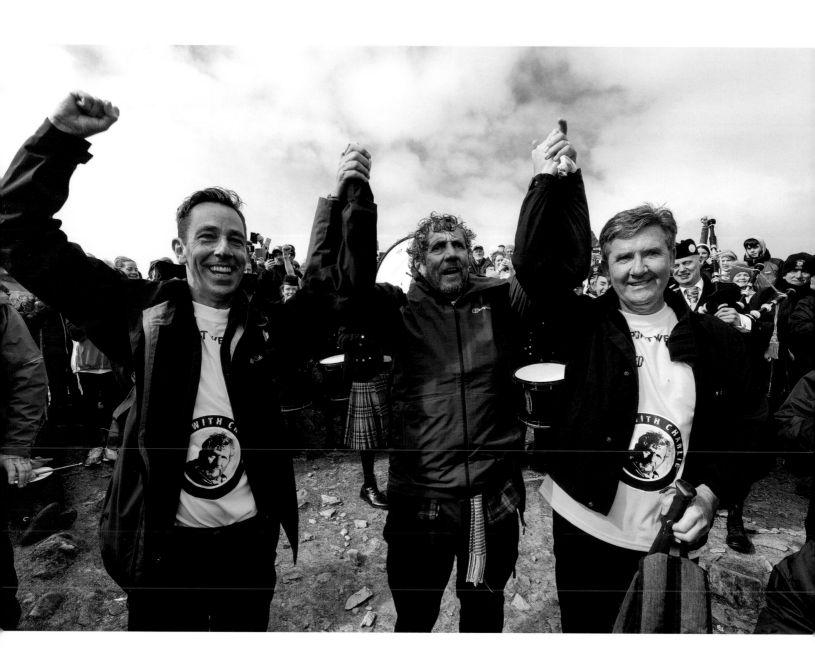

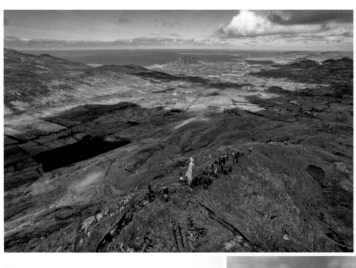
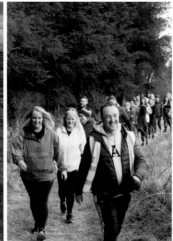
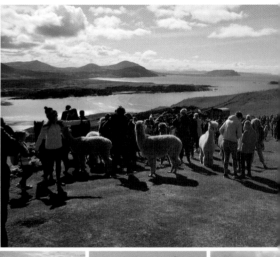
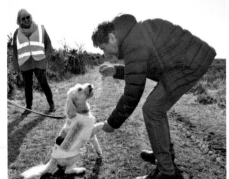
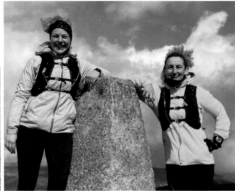
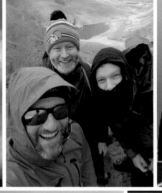
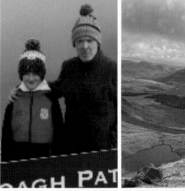
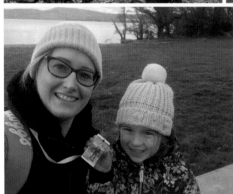
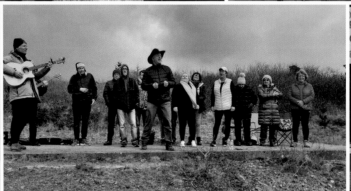
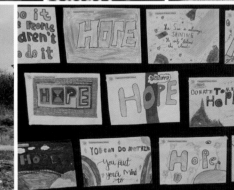
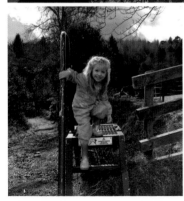
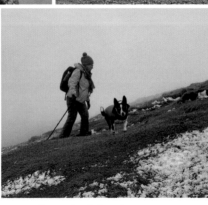
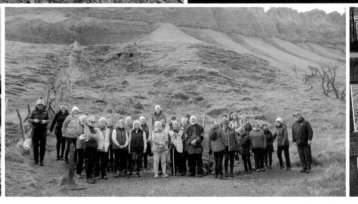

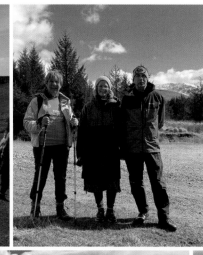
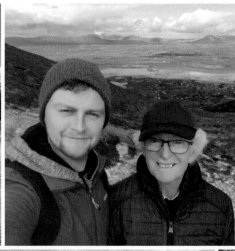
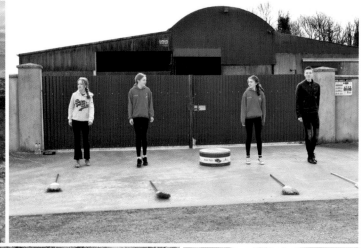
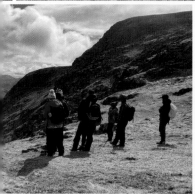
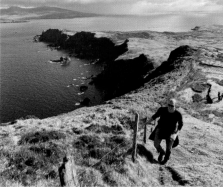
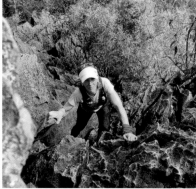
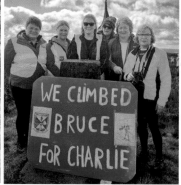
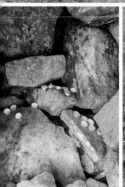
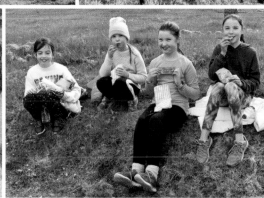
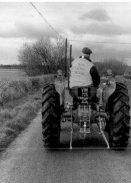
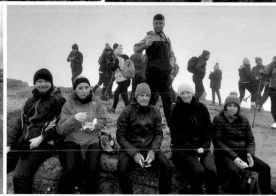
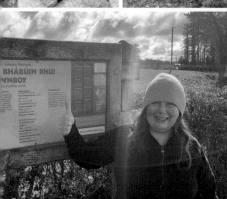
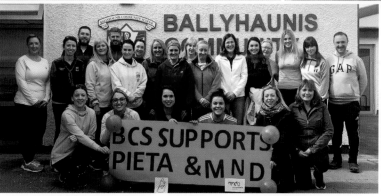
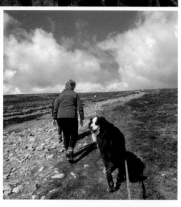

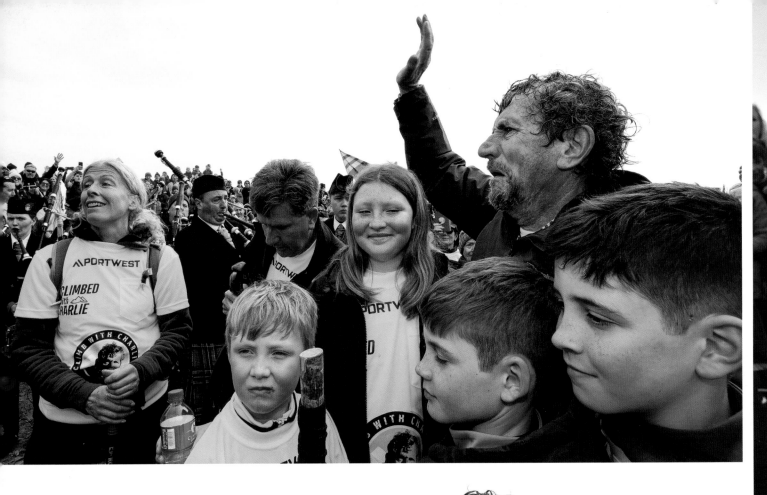
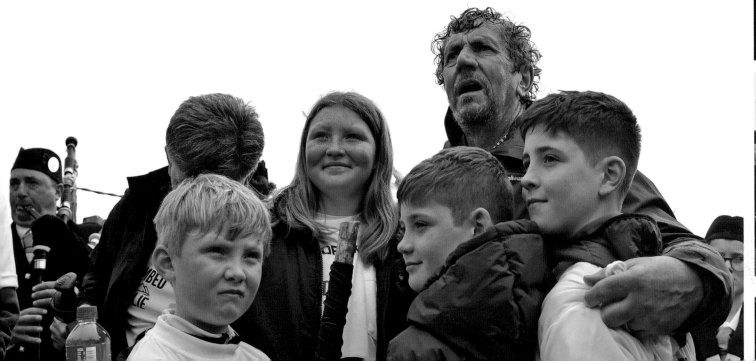

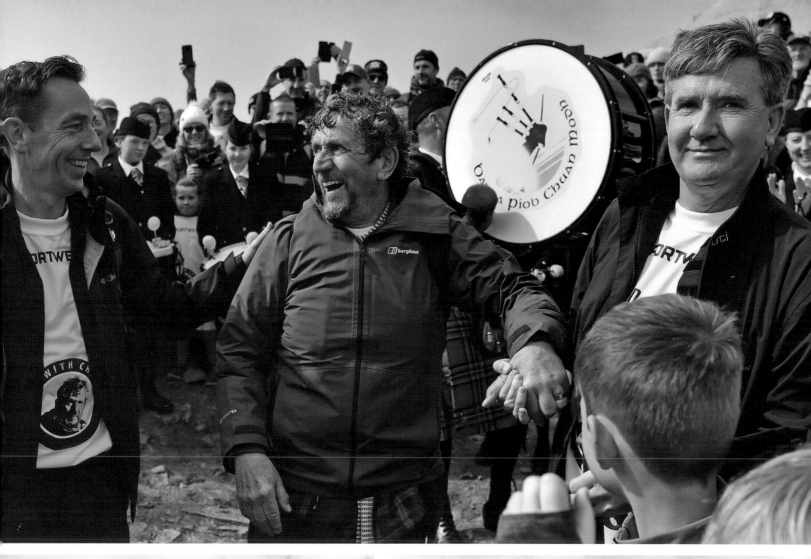

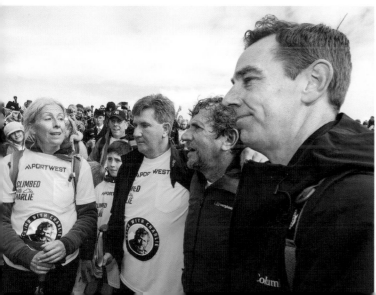

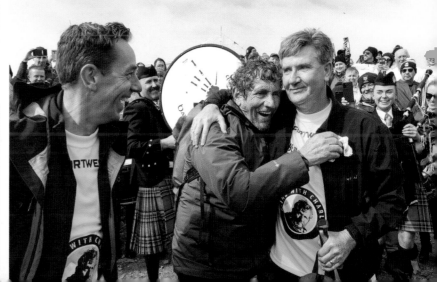

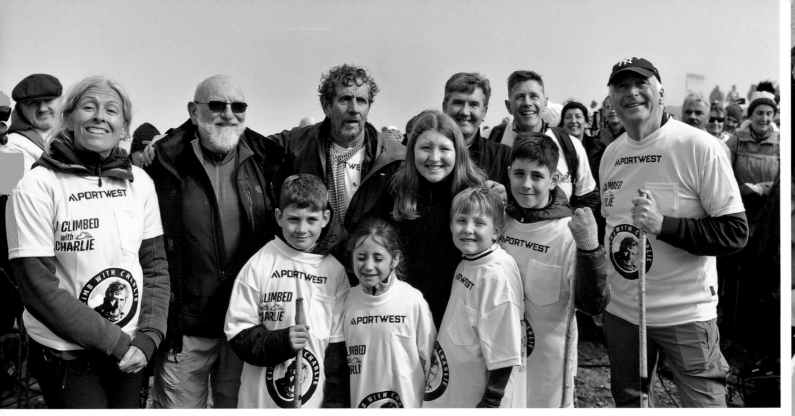

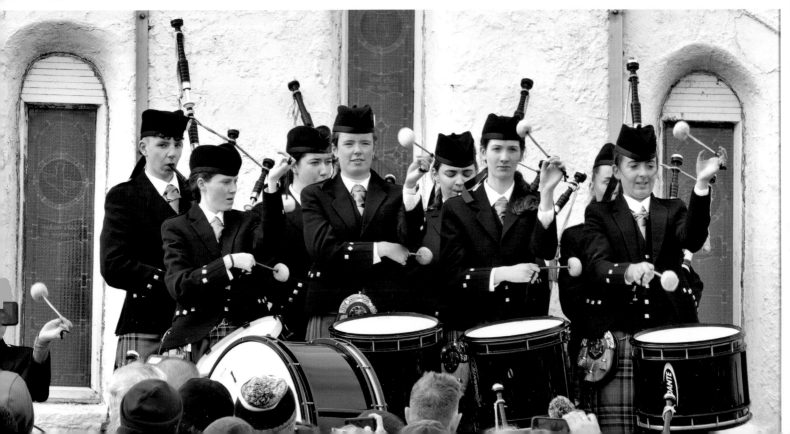

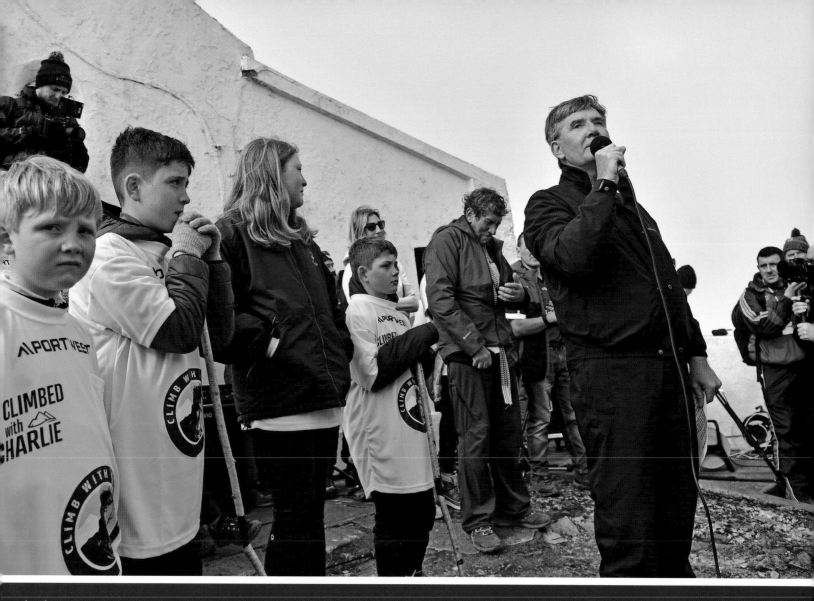

Climb With Charlie was an event that will live in my memory for as long as I live. To stand at the bottom of Croagh Patrick and look up and see the thousands of people making their way up the mountain and feel the sense of community and togetherness was amazing. To eventually stand at the top, shoulder to shoulder with Charlie and Claire while the Clew Bay Band played so beautifully, was one of the most emotional experiences I've ever had. I feel privileged and honoured to have been a part of something so special. Thank you, Charlie, you are an incredible human being.

Daniel O'Donnell

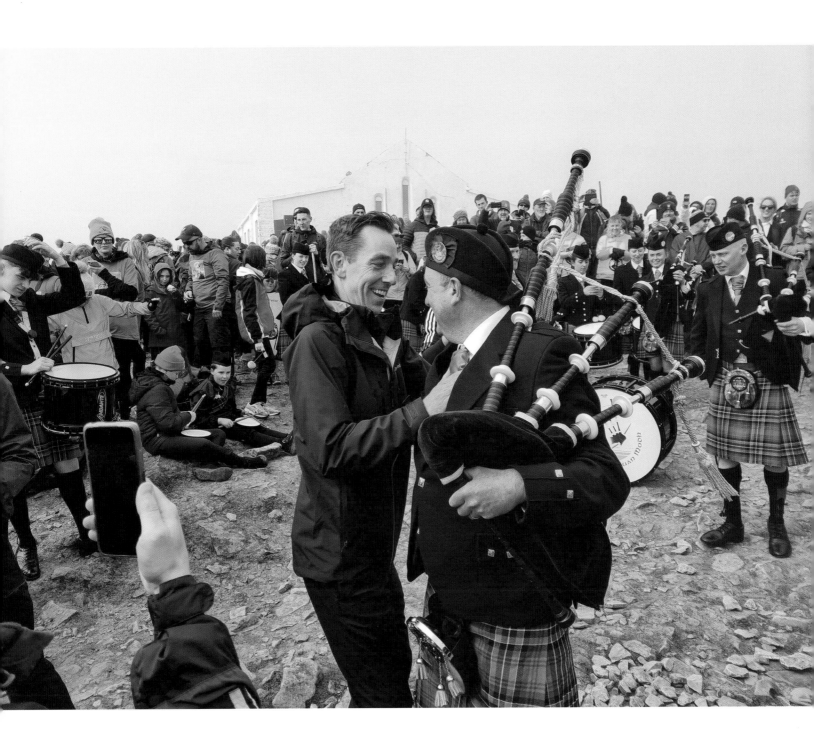

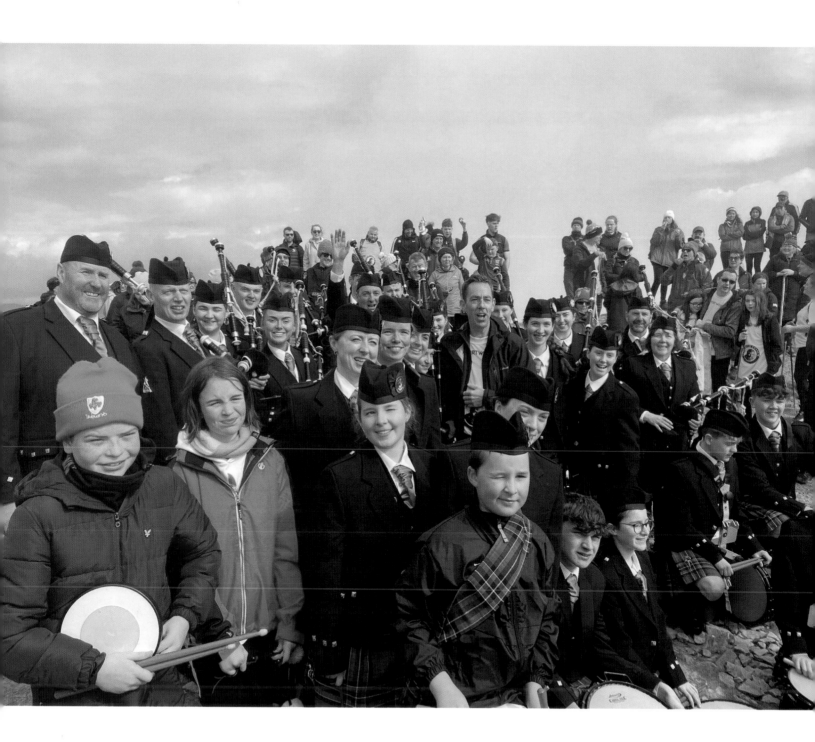

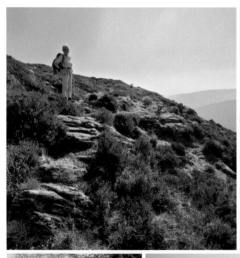
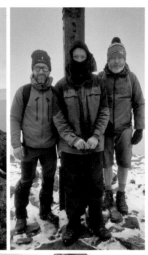
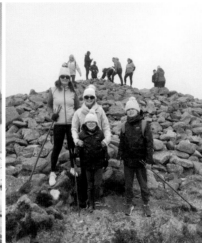
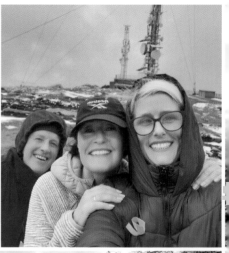
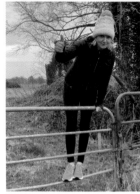
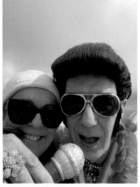
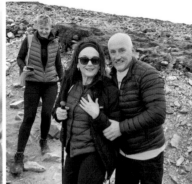
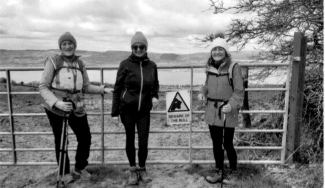
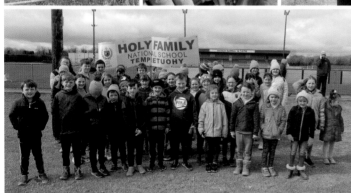
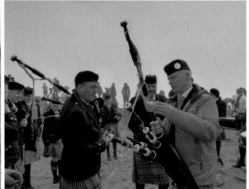
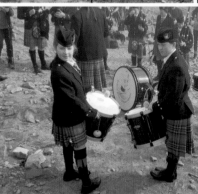
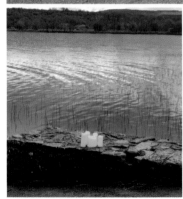
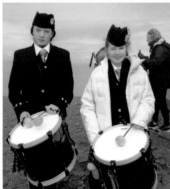
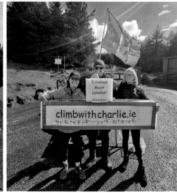
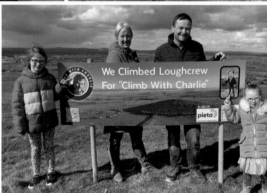

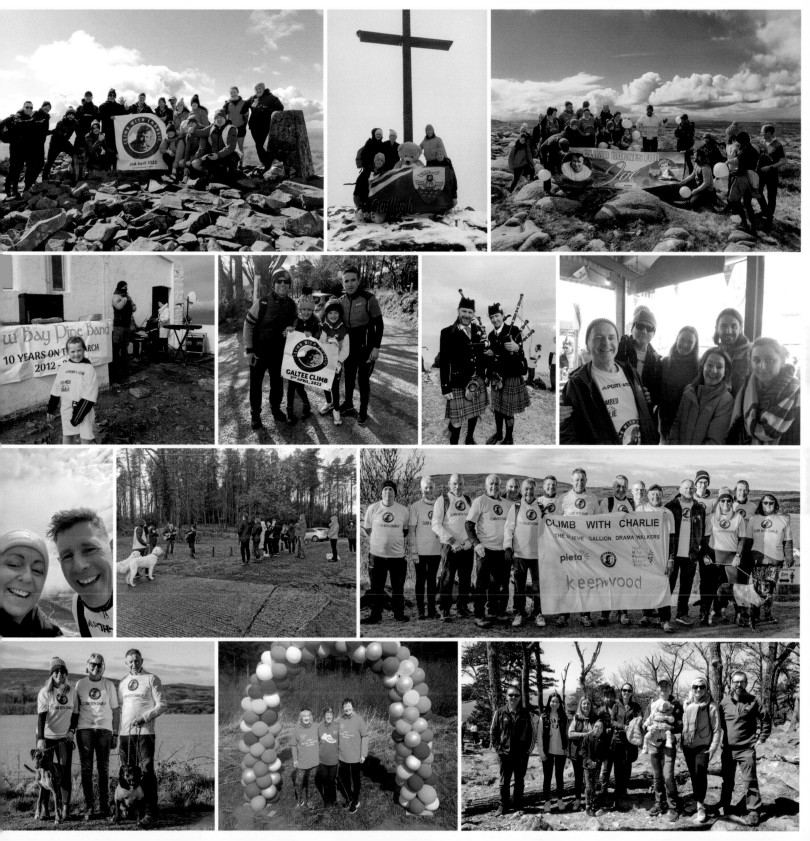

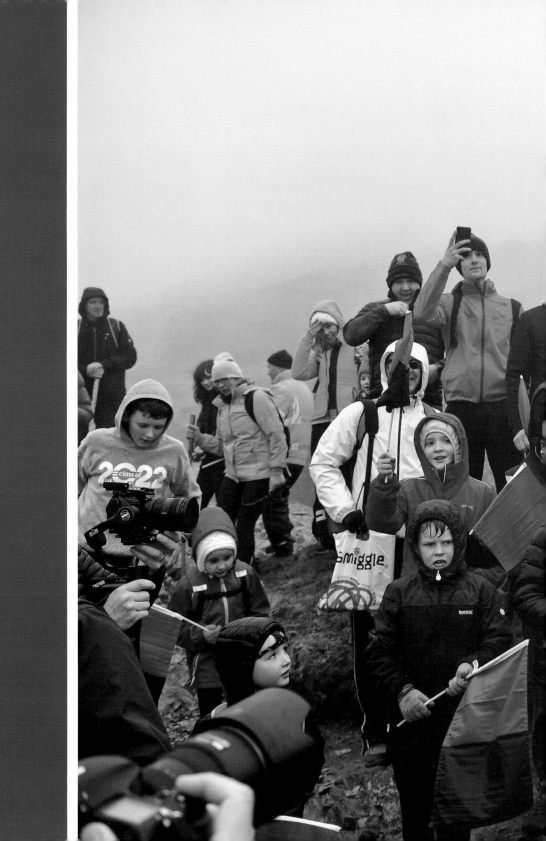

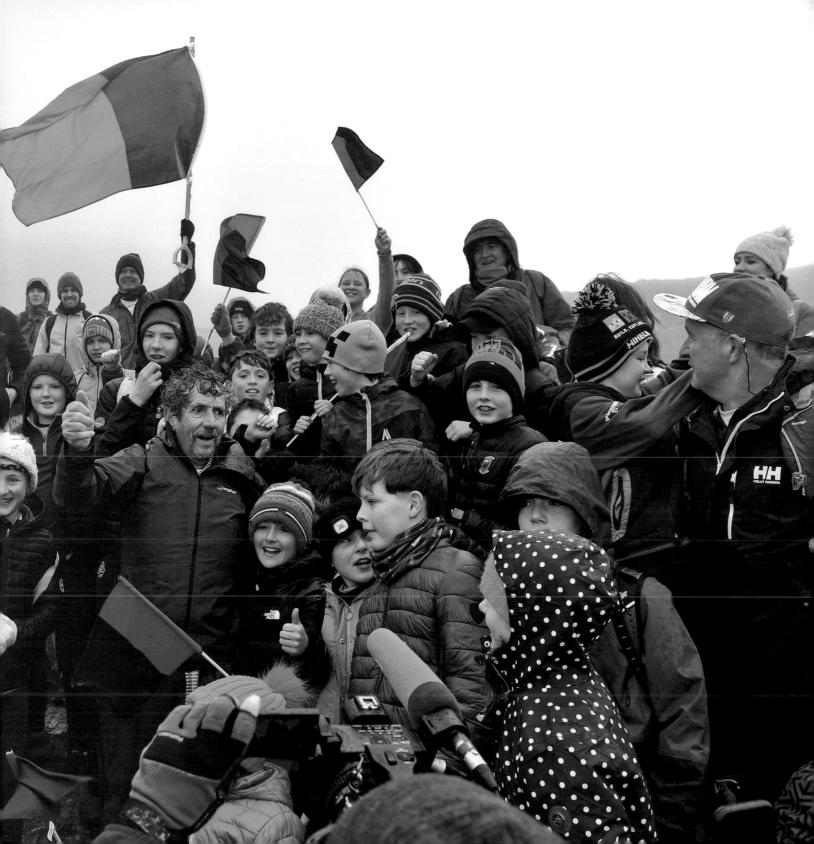

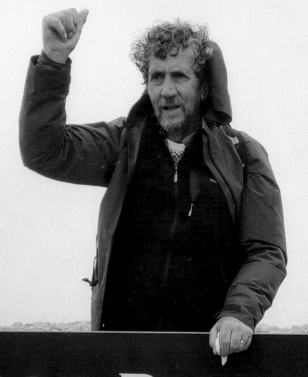

CROAGH PATRICK
IRELAND'S HOLY MOUNTAIN

CRUACH PHÁDRAIG
SLIABH NAOFA NA HÉIREANN

 WWW.WESTPORTPARISH.IE

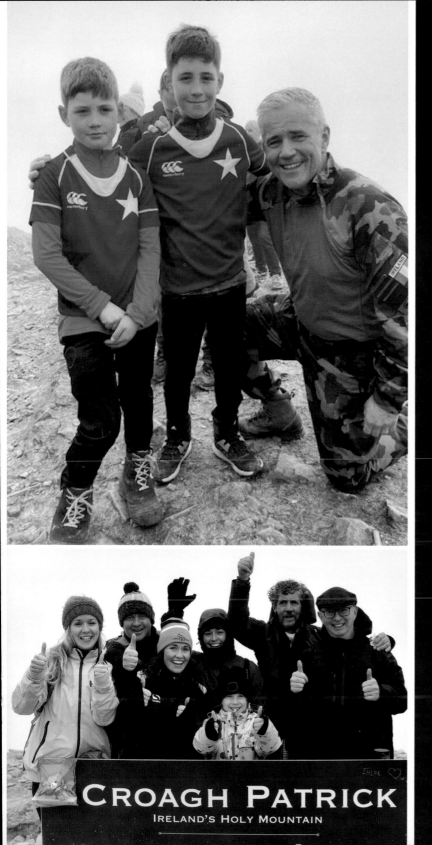

The 2nd of April 2022 will remain etched in my memory forever. Climb With Charlie presented us all with the opportunity of being 'present', that is, to be in the moment.

The climb brought us together as a community where we were able to appreciate each other and witness the best of humanity, to celebrate the simplicity and the joy of life.

Sometimes I found myself falling into step on the climb with strangers, yet everyone was a friend, everyone was chatting, everyone had a smile and everyone had a sense of being part of something really special, we were all truly 'present'.

It was a privilege to be part of this climb, a day that will no doubt transcend time and live with us all in our memory as a day that was, quite simply, special.

Thank you, Charlie.

Seán Clancy
Lieutenant General
Chief of Staff
Irish Defence Forces

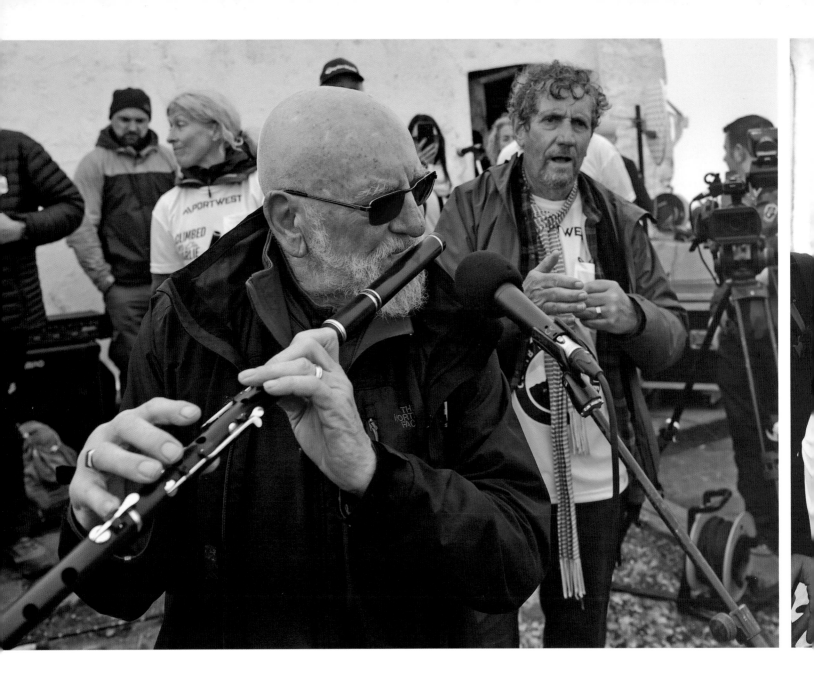

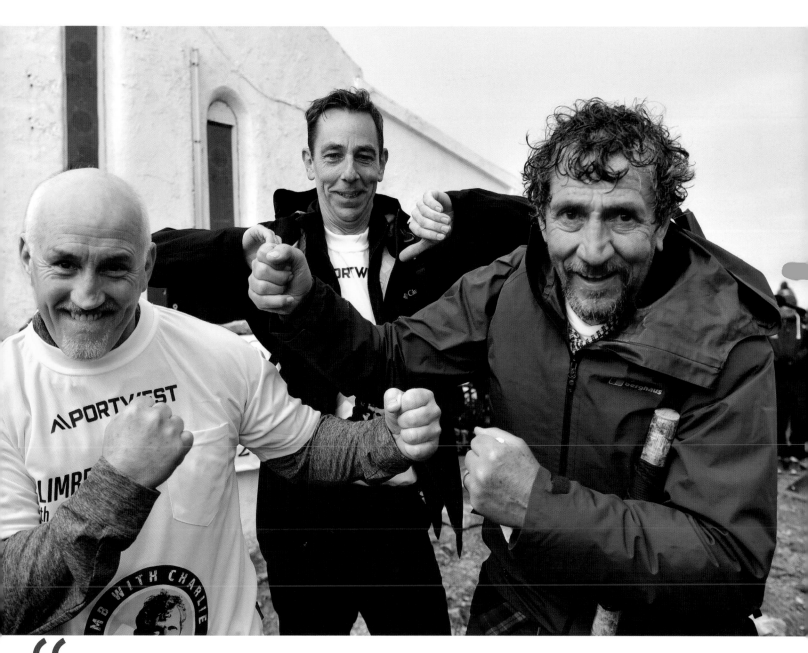

It was an honour to Climb With Charlie up Croagh Patrick. I spend my time in the boxing business, where I see men and women showing mental strength and determination to achieve their objectives, but rarely have I witnessed the type of courage and commitment that Charlie Bird showed on 2 April to get up and down that mountain. Charlie, I salute you.

Barry McGuigan

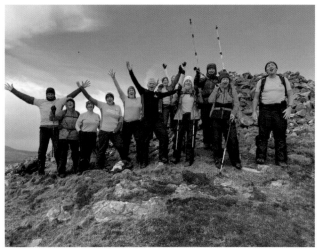
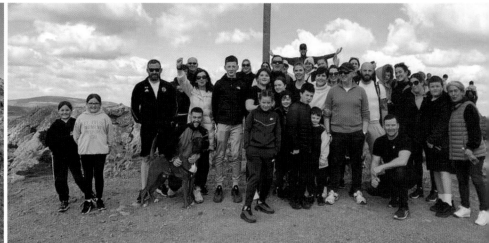
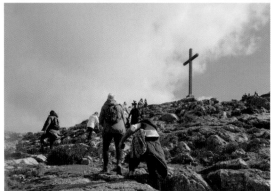
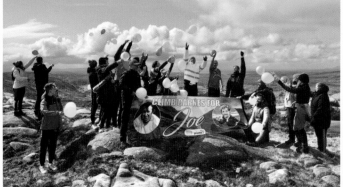
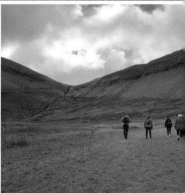
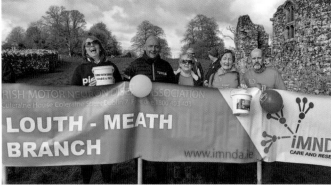
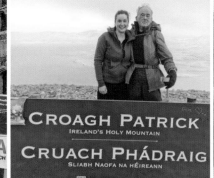
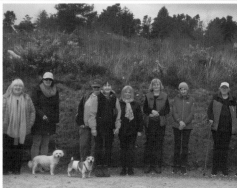

LOUTH - MEATH
BRANCH

CROAGH PATRICK
IRELAND'S HOLY MOUNTAIN

CRUACH PHÁDRAIG
SLIABH NAOFA NA HÉIREANN

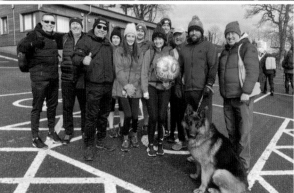
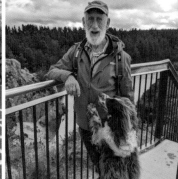
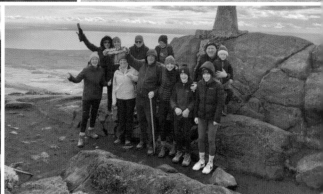

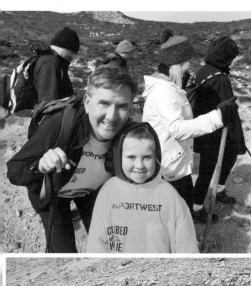
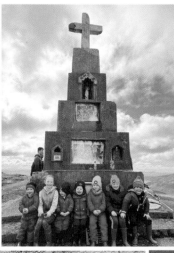
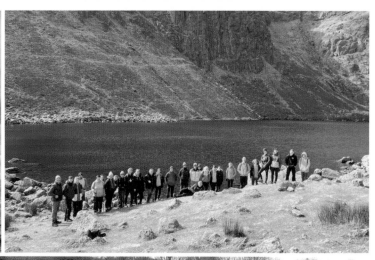
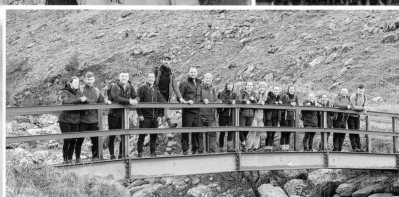
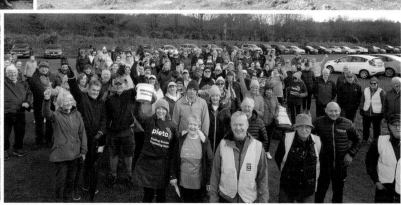
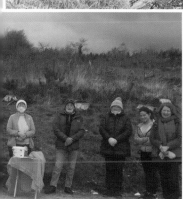
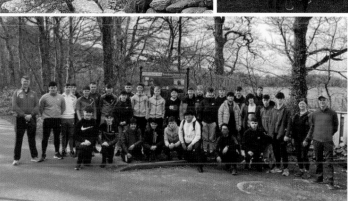
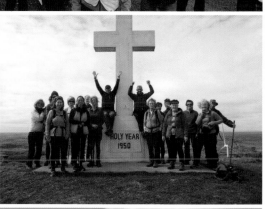
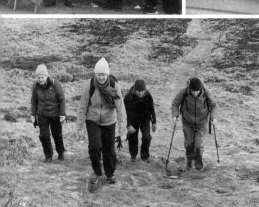
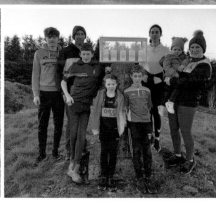
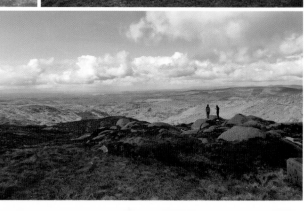

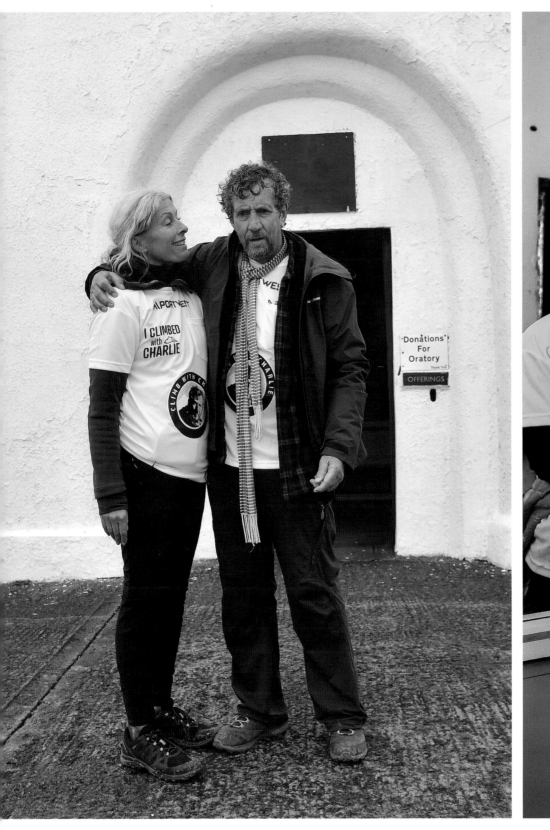
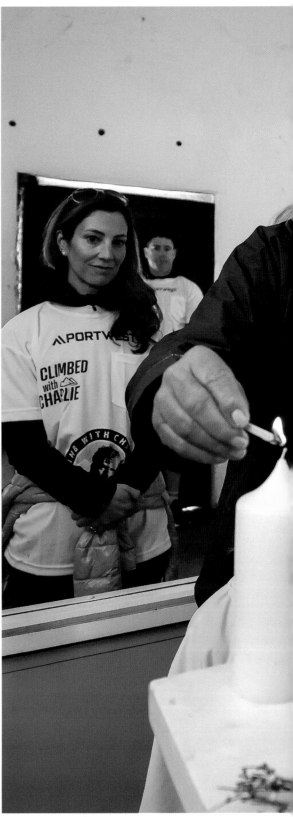

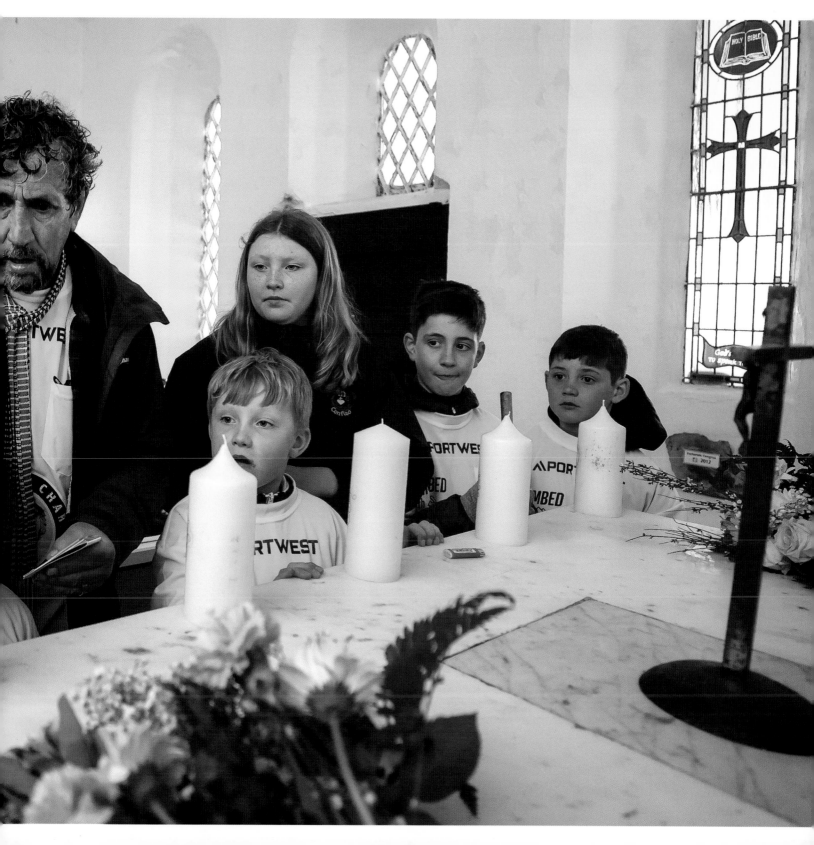

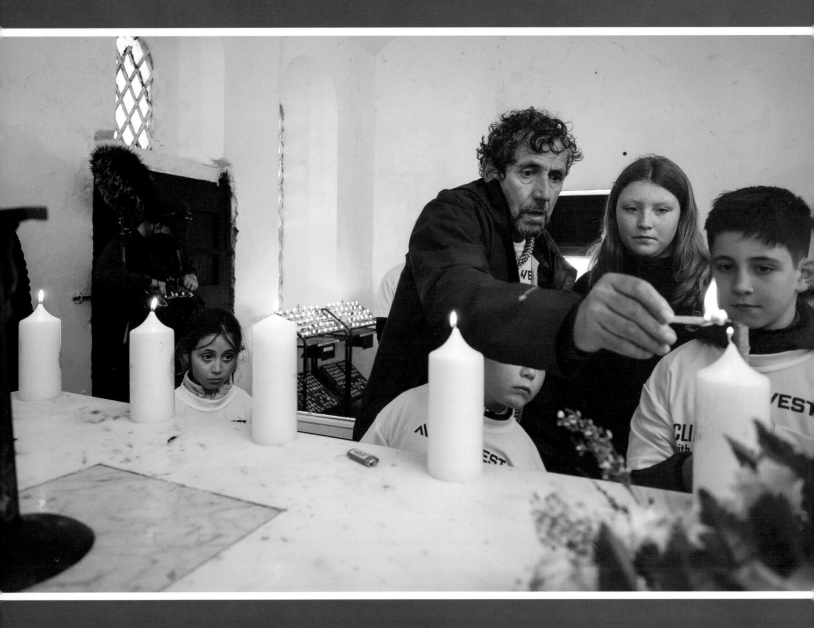

CHARLIE'S FIVE CANDLES

Candle One:
For Vicky Phelan

Candle Two:
For those with a
terminal illness

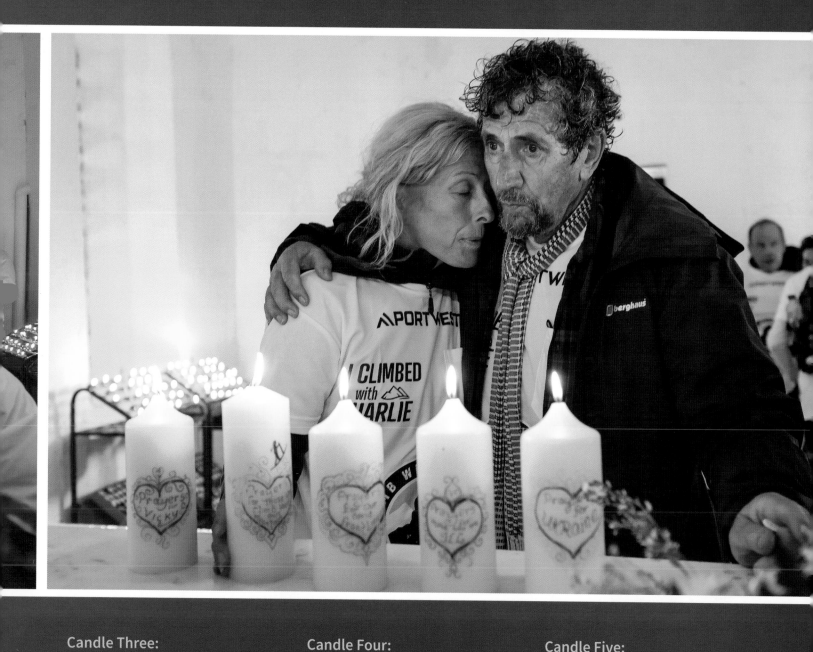

Candle Three:
For those in a dark place, climbing their own personal mountains

Candle Four:
To celebrate everyone who worked so hard to help in the battle against the pandemic

Candle Five:
For the people of Ukraine

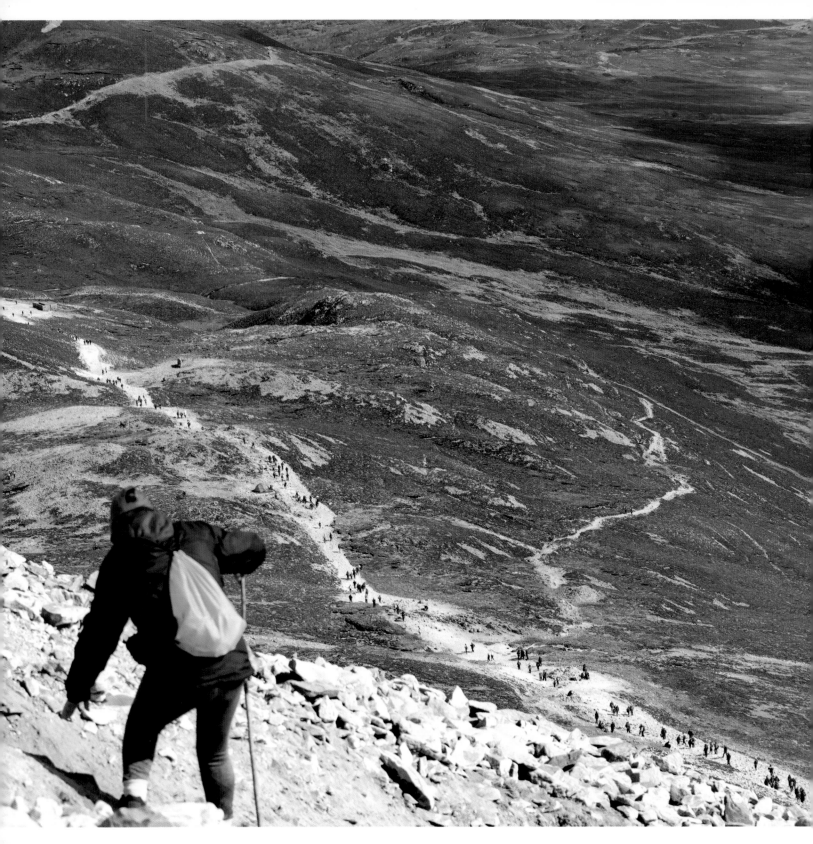

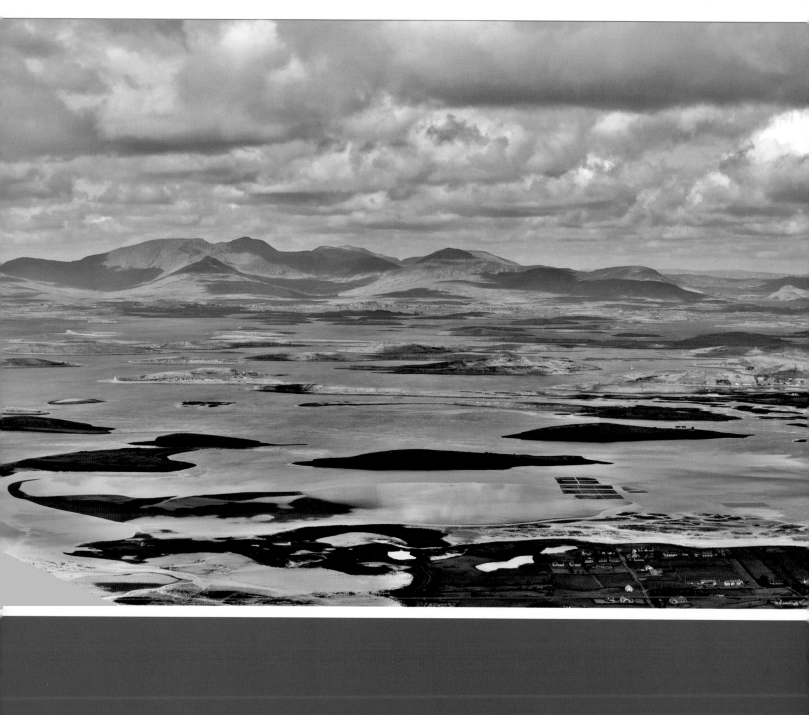

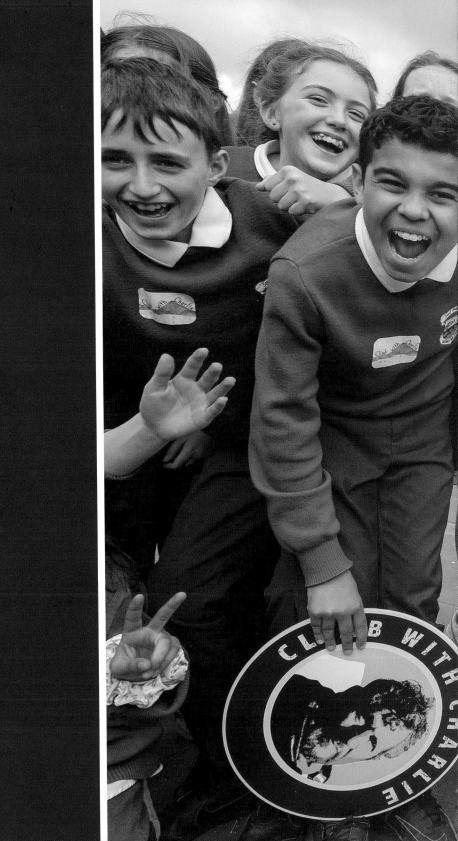

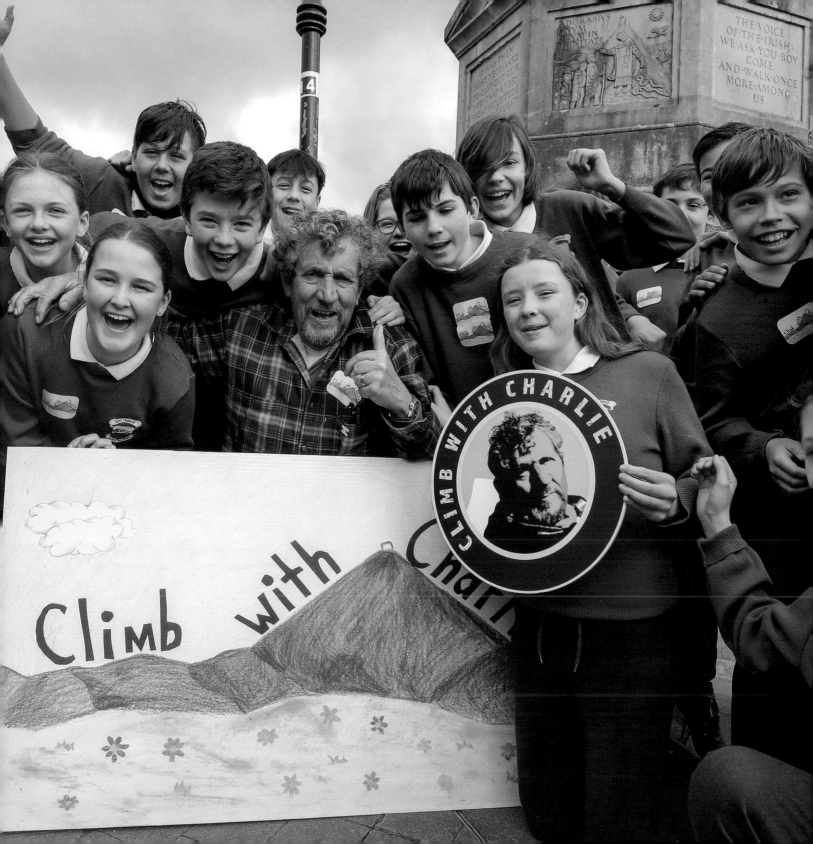

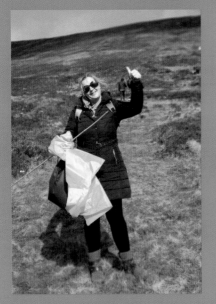

OUR DEEPEST SYMPATHY to the family and friends of Cora O'Grady, who took ill and sadly passed away on 2 April while out climbing Galtymore Mountain for Climb With Charlie.

A special word of thanks is due to the amazing volunteers of the South Eastern Mountain Rescue Team, who took such good care of Cora on the mountain.

THANK YOU FROM CHARLIE

I WOULD LIKE TO THANK the Climb With Charlie team for all their efforts: Paul Allen, Claire Corbett, Denise Cronin, Kerry Fitzgerald, Sarah Joyce, Lillian McGovern, Rory Sweeney and Gemma Watts. These people have worked so hard and I'm so grateful to them.

I would also like to say a special word of thanks to Fr Charlie McDonnell and Denis Harrington, who both played such a key role in helping to organise the climb.

Finally, I would like to thank my wonderful wife Claire for all her support and hard work on the climb and on this beautiful book.

PHOTO CREDITS

Key to images: bottom (b); top (t); left (l); right (r)

Mark Condren: 51 (t); **Karen Cox:** 21, 35 (bl), 45 (b), 48 (t, br); **Dee Forbes:** 18, 20 (br), 24, 32, 34 (tl), 76, 82, 83 (t); **Conor McKeown:** 27, 33, 34 (t, br), 35 (t), 50 (tr), 51 (bl), 56, 57, 58, 66–7, 72 (b), 73 (t), 74 (t), 75, 80–1, 83 (t, br), 83 (b), 84, 85, 88; **Michael Mc Laughlin:** 20 (t); **Gerry Mooney:** 11, 49, 50 (tl, b), 51 (br), 52–3, 61 (t, br), 64, 68, 69, 72 (t), 73 (bl, br), 89, 90, 91, 94–5; **Padraig O'Reilly:** 8, 25, 26, 28, 35 (br), 61 (bl); **Brendan St John:** 15, 16, 17, 19, 36, 37, 40, 41, 42, 43, 44, 45 (t), 48 (bl), 59, 60, 65, 74 (b), 92, 93

We would like to thank everyone who contributed to this book by sending in pictures of their own Climb With Charlie. Many of these people had their own personal challenges and mountains to climb, so it is lovely to include their photographs in the book.

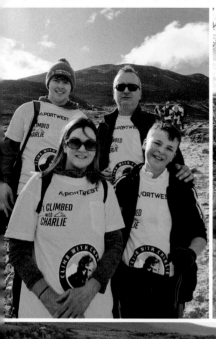
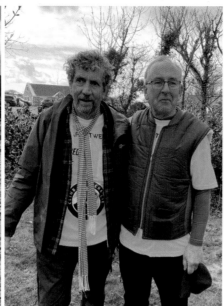
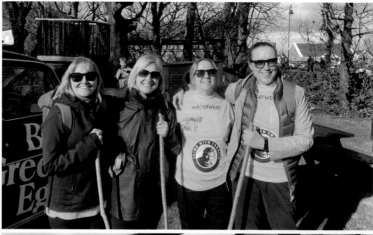
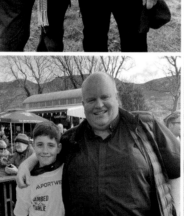
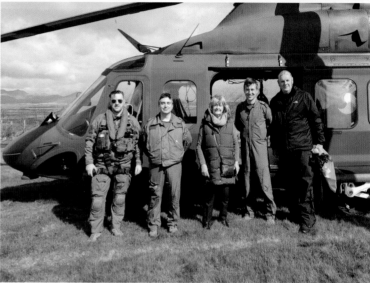
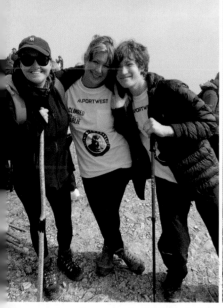
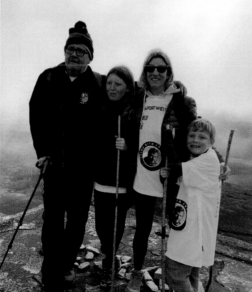
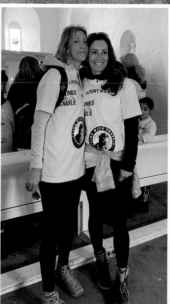
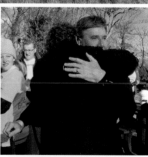
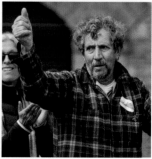

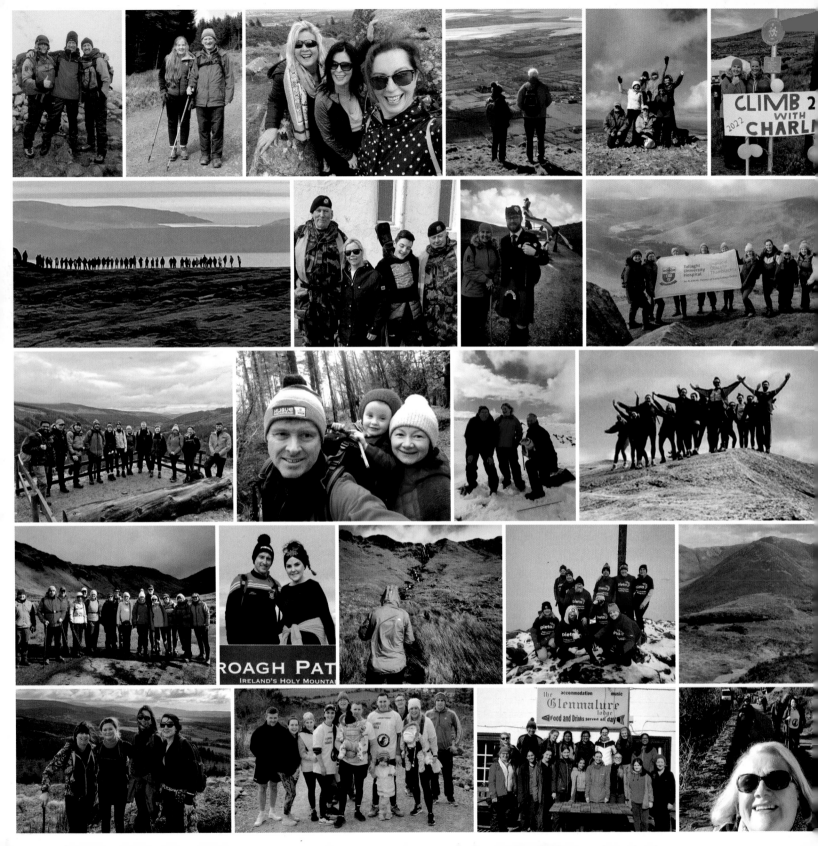